Heart Care for Life

A Yale University Press Health & Wellness book is an authoritative, accessible source of information on a health-related topic. It may provide guidance to help you lead a healthy life, examine your treatment options for a specific condition or disease, situate a healthcare issue in the context of your life as a whole, or address questions or concerns that linger after visits to your healthcare provider.

Thomas E. Brown, Ph.D., *Attention Deficit Disorder: The Unfocused Mind in Children and Adults*

Ruth Grobstein, M.D., Ph.D., *The Breast Cancer Book: What You Need to Know to Make Informed Decisions*

James Hicks, M.D., *Fifty Signs of Mental Illness: A Guide to Understanding Mental Health*

Mary Jane Minkin, M.D., and Carol V. Wright, Ph.D., *A Woman's Guide to Menopause and Perimenopause*

Mary Jane Minkin, M.D., and Carol V. Wright, Ph.D., *A Woman's Guide to Sexual Health*

Catherine M. Poole, with DuPont Guerry IV, M.D., *Melanoma: Prevention, Detection, and Treatment,* 2nd ed.

Barry L. Zaret, M.D., and Genell J. Subak-Sharpe, M.S., *Heart Care for Life: Developing the Program That Works Best for You*

HEART CARE FOR LIFE

Developing
the Program That
Works Best for You

Barry L. Zaret, M.D.
Genell J. Subak-Sharpe, M.S.

YALE UNIVERSITY PRESS/NEW HAVEN & LONDON

The information and suggestions contained in this book are not intended to replace the services of your physician or caregiver. Because each person and each medical situation is unique, you should consult your own physician to get answers to your personal questions, to evaluate any symptoms you may have, or to receive suggestions on appropriate medications.

The authors have attempted to make this book as accurate and up to date as possible, but it may nevertheless contain errors, omissions, or material that is out of date at the time you read it. Neither the authors nor the publisher has any legal responsibility or liability for errors, omissions, out-of-date material, or the reader's application of the medical information or advice contained in this book.

Designed by Mary Valencia.
Set in Minion type by Integrated Publishing Solutions.
Printed in the United States of America by Vail-Ballou Press.

Library of Congress Cataloging-in-Publication Data

Zaret, Barry L.
    Heart care for life : developing the program that works best for you / Barry L. Zaret, Genell J. Subak-Sharpe.
        p.   cm.
    Includes bibliographical references and index.
    ISBN-13: 978-0-300-10869-9 (alk. paper)
    ISBN-10: 0-300-10869-9 (alk. paper)
    1. Heart—Diseases—Popular works. 2. Heart—Diseases—Prevention—Popular works. I. Subak-Sharpe, Genell J. II. Title.
RC672.Z35 2006
616.1'205—dc22   2005023367

A catalogue record for this book is available from the British Library.

The paper in this book meets the guidelines for permanence and durability of the Committee on Production Guidelines for Book Longevity of the Council on Library Resources.

10 9 8 7 6 5 4 3 2 1

*To the many patients whose need for individualized cardiac care
has provided a framework for ideas presented in this book.
You have taught as well as received.*

CONTENTS

List of Abbreviations   **ix**

Preface   **xi**

Introduction   **xvi**

1. A Personalized Plan: The Key to a Lifelong Heart Program   **1**

    PART I: LIFESTYLE AND HEART HEALTH   **25**

2. Exercise Your Way to a Healthy Heart and Body   **31**

3. Adopting a Heart-Healthy Diet   **50**

4. Stress, Depression, and Other Psychological Factors   **69**

5. Controlling and Stopping Smoking   **82**

    PART II: THE BASICS OF LIFELONG TREATMENT   **93**

6. Diagnostic Tests and Procedures   **97**

7. Treating Your Heart Condition   **120**

8. Alternative and Complementary Therapies   **154**

    PART III: POPULATIONS WITH SPECIAL
    CONCERNS   **165**

9. Heart Care for Women   **169**

10. Heart Disease in the Elderly   **179**

11. Heart Disease in Minority Populations 186

12. Young Athletes and Heart Disease 192

13. Adults with Congenital Heart Disease 199

14. Practical Advice for Travelers 206

PART IV: ADVANCES IN TREATING HEART DISEASE
AND HOPE FOR THE FUTURE 213

15. Recently Developed Devices and Procedures 217

16. Biologically Based Therapies 228

17. Experimental Treatments and Clinical Trials 239

Epilogue 244

Acknowledgments 246

Glossary 247

Further Reading and Resources 256

Index 261

A B B R E V I A T I O N S

ABI	Ankle/brachial index	EPC	Endothelial progenitor cells
ACE	Angiotensin converting inhibitor enzyme inhibitor	EPS	Electrophysiological testing
		ERNA	equilibrium radionuclide angiocardiography
ACS	Acute coronary syndrome		
AED	Automated external defibrillator	FDA	Food and Drug Administration
AHA	American Heart Association	FGF	Fibroblast growth factor
		HACE	High-altitude cerebral edema
AMA	American Medical Association	HAPE	High-altitude pulmonary edema
AMS	Acute mountain sickness		
ARBs	Angiotensin receptor blockers	HCM	Hypertrophic cardiomyopathy
ASBS	American Society for Bariatric Surgery	HDL	High-density lipoprotein
		HRT	Hormone replacement therapy
AV node	Atrioventricular node		
BMI	Body mass index	hs-CRP	High-sensitivity C-reactive protein test
CABG	Coronary artery bypass graft		
		ICD	Implanted cardiac defibrillator
CAD	Coronary artery disease		
CRP	C-reactive protein	IHSS	Idiopathic hypertrophic subaortic stenosis
CRT	Cardiac resynchronization therapy		
		IVUS	Intravascular ultrasound
CT	Computed tomography	LDL	Low-density lipoprotein
ECG/EKG	Electrocardiogram	Lp(a)	Lipoprotein (a)
EECP	Enhanced external counterpulsation	METs	Metabolic equivalents
		MI	Myocardial infarction

MRA	Magnetic resonance angiography	PPH	Primary pulmonary hypertension
MRI	Magnetic resonance imaging	PTCA	Percutaneous transluminal coronary angioplasty
MUGA	Multigated acquisition scan	PVD	Peripheral vascular disease
NHANES	National Health and Nutrition Examination Survey	SPECT	Single photon emission computed tomography
PCI	Percutaneous coronary intervention	SSRI	Selective serotonin receptor inhibitor
PET	Positron emission tomography	TEE	Transesophageal echocardiography
PFO	Patent foramen ovale	VAD	Ventricular assist device
PPCM	Peripartum cardiomyopathy	VEGF	Vascular endothelial growth factor

PREFACE

This book is based on concepts that have evolved over thirty-five years of personally caring for heart patients. Our goal throughout is to help you become a meaningful partner in the management of your own cardiovascular care. We provide a wealth of information on the diagnosis and treatment of different forms of heart disease. But equally important, you'll find a blueprint for making small lifestyle changes that can make the difference between a shortened life marked by increasing disability and a longer, productive one that allows you to enjoy normal daily activities.

Our approach both emphasizes the need for individualized care and offers advice that will benefit all readers as they begin a new journey toward better heart health. From this book, you will learn that

💜 To become an empowered patient, you must enter into a meaningful relationship with your health-care provider that defines your role in maintaining your health.

💜 You and your health-care providers need to tailor any treatment strategy or lifestyle change to your particular needs.

💜 If you are to take your own health seriously, you must make permanent lifestyle changes based on understanding. These changes cannot be based on fear, panic, or unreasonableness, and they must be combined with state-of-the-art medical therapy to achieve optimal results.

💜 Although there is seldom a cure for cardiovascular disease, virtually all patients can be helped. Ongoing scientific and technical advances provide ample reason for meaningful hope, even if you are afflicted with serious heart problems.

Although cardiovascular disease remains the leading cause of death in the United States, the toll has been cut in half over the last forty years, thanks to tremendous medical and scientific advances. Even so, statistics from the American Heart Association show that cardiovascular diseases claimed an estimated 932,000 American lives in 2002—the latest year for which mortality statistics are available—accounting for about 38 percent of all deaths. Clearly, much work remains to be done. Again, to cite statistics released by the American Heart Association in 2005:

- More than 70 million Americans—one out of every five—have one or more forms of cardiovascular disease.
- Sudden cardiac death—defined as death before a person can be hospitalized—claims about 335,000 lives a year. Most of these deaths are due to a cardiac arrest caused by ventricular fibrillation, a devastating disturbance in the heart's normal rhythm.
- More than 13 million Americans suffer from coronary artery disease (CAD); of these, more than 6 million suffer from bouts of chest pain (angina pectoris).
- More than 7 million Americans a year have a heart attack (also known by its medical term myocardial infarction, or MI).
- More than 65 million Americans have high blood pressure, putting them at increased risk for heart attack, heart failure, stroke, kidney failure, peripheral vascular disease, and other serious complications.
- More than 5 million Americans suffer a stroke each year.
- The American Heart Association estimates that the total cost of cardiovascular disease in the United States will exceed $393 billion in 2005.

Although most cardiovascular deaths occur in people over the age of sixty-five, many thousands are struck down during the prime of life. Sudden, unexpected death from a cardiac arrest occurs at an average age of sixty, just when most individuals are at peak productivity. Thousands of others die at even earlier ages, leaving behind young children.

Consequently, the fundamental importance of cardiovascular care in the context of total health care cannot be overemphasized. We, as individuals, need to learn how we can either prevent heart disease or seek out the most effective approach to treatment should it develop. Over the past decade a large number of publications, varying from the straightforward to the sensational, have dealt with heart disease treatment and prevention. Myriad "breakthrough" diet regimens have been devised, only to be debunked by advances in research. Other "revolutions" have advocated strict approaches to lifestyle, suitable only for a monk living in mountain isolation. Sadly, such fads come and go without really changing the long-term outlook of heart patients or those at risk of developing cardiovascular disease. This book was conceived with a twofold purpose: to articulate a thoughtful philosophy of patient care and self-care that has evolved over more than three decades, and to describe the great advances that promise to save countless lives and improve the quality of life for persons with even very severe heart disease.

Throughout, we emphasize the need for personalized, lifelong programs for heart patients. The one-size-fits-all strategy has never been viable: instead we propose a rational approach that leads to long-term benefits, consistency, and awareness, and combines both the art and the science of clinical medicine. This is an approach that you, together with your physician when appropriate, can use to develop a lifelong program that fits your lifestyle and meets your medical needs.

A fundamental part of this approach (and, for that matter, any approach to medical care) is the empowerment of individuals to assume an active role—and responsibility—in their care. It is not enough to leave your care to your doctor, and you won't get far if you assume a "don't tell me, I don't want to know" attitude. Instead, take the time to learn about your condition, to ask your caregivers relevant questions, and to take part in the design of a lifelong program based on your individual needs, problems, and variables.

Above all, it's essential to remember that there are no quick fixes. The individualized program must be adopted as a lifelong (and life-sustaining) endeavor. Although the idea of no quick fixes seems obvious, all too often it does not represent current everyday life or medical care. How many individuals have thrown up their hands in frustration when a diet "failed" or an exercise program resulted in injury? How many times have setbacks resulted in a medical program being abandoned rather than modified? In a lifelong plan, a setback is viewed simply as a bump in the road, instead of its end. Rather than impatience and frustration, a lifelong approach leads to flexibility, modification, the frequent rethinking of issues, and a meaningful interaction with your physician.

For the most part, medical professionals don't *cure* cardiovascular disease; rather, they modify it, modulate it, and treat it within a specific context. Cardiovascular disease is not like an inflamed appendix or a straightforward bacterial pneumonia, which can be cured through appropriate treatment. Instead, it is usually a progressive condition that takes years to develop, is multifaceted in origin, and will require attention for the rest of your life. The earlier you accept and act on these facts, the better. All too often, doctors encounter patients with severely advanced disease and problems that could have been forestalled with earlier intervention. Such a "wait and see" attitude by the patient or caregiver is dangerous. There's no such thing as "a touch of diabetes" or "mild high blood pressure," implying that early stages of these disorders are so insignificant that they can be ignored. Instead there is ample evidence that early, aggressive treatment of high blood pressure, diabetes, and other documented abnormalities can halt or delay progression, whereas "watchful waiting" often results in irreversible damage and a shortened life.

All forms of cardiovascular disease must be dealt with rationally, sensibly, and not entirely out of fear. Fear may initially motivate an individual to adopt a major new therapeutic program, but it invariably recedes over time; it cannot sustain a successful program of lifelong lifestyle change.

This book emphasizes the delicate balance between the core medical values—the parameters doctors use to determine risk and devise a treatment plan—and the individual variables that define *personalized* patient care. Core values form the constants of cardiovascular health and include issues related to medical and surgical therapy, obesity, diet, exercise, stress, smoking, and various forms of diagnostic testing. Variables comprise the individual differences that define specific patients and are critical in developing a workable lifelong heart-care program. Although these concepts seem obvious, they are seldom fully appreciated in actual medical practice today.

It is not wrong to be different. Current medical practice is based on evidence derived from large patient populations. Extrapolating those data to an individual's situation is always risky. Genetics are a major factor accounting for this variability. We all have very different biochemistries. Slight differences in specific enzymes can lead to major differences in the occurrence and manifestation of disease. These differences help explain why some people respond well to a certain drug or treatment, while in others the same medication is ineffective or even toxic. Indeed, many drugs in current use are effective in fewer than 40 percent of patients. This realization is prompting a whole new science of pharmacogenomics, based on genetic differences and how individuals deal with drugs. Statistical analysis determines whether the benefits of the drugs outweigh their potential liabilities in large populations. Statistics, however, do not address whether an individual will be treated effectively or have unpredictable major side effects.

The same individualized, targeted approach is needed for all aspects of cardiovascular care. For example, a diet that does not take into account individual tastes, food preferences, and eating habits is generally a waste of time and effort. Socioeconomic status, education, presence of other diseases (comorbidity), occupation, interaction with one's spouse and family, and many other individual factors also affect the success of any treatment. As a patient, it is not your responsibility to adjust your life to a one-size-fits-all plan. Rather, it is the joint responsibility of the patient, the medical practitioner, and the health-care system to work together to design a program that fits the individual.

Finally, every patient in a long-term care program needs hope based on rational thought and understanding. As Dr. Jerome Groopman stated in his 2003 book *The Anatomy of Hope:*

> Hope is one of our central emotions and we are often at a loss when asked to define it. Many of us confuse hope with optimism, a prevailing attitude that "things turn out for the best." But hope differs from optimism. Hope does not arise from being told to "think positively" or from hearing an overly rosy forecast. Hope, unlike optimism, is rooted in unalloyed reality. . . . Hope is the elevating feeling we experience when we see—in the mind's eye—a path to a better future. Hope acknowledges the significant obstacles and deep pitfalls along that path. True hope has no room for delusion. Clearly, hope gives us the courage to confront our circumstances and the capacity to surmount them. For all my patients, hope, true hope, has proved as important as any medication I might prescribe or any procedure that I might perform. Only well into my career did I come to realize this.

Indeed there is substantial reason for heart patients to feel hopeful. The past several decades have brought enormous strides in cardiovascular care. Patients are now surviving conditions that would have proved fatal only a few years ago. Heart attacks can be stopped, or their damage limited, if they are treated within an hour or two of their occurrence. In the catheterization laboratory, we can now open blocked coronary arteries causing the attack or administer clot-dissolving drugs to restore blood flow before major heart damage occurs. New medications are leading to major advances in heart-disease prevention, to improvements in symptoms when heart disease is already present, and to changes in the basic biology of the disease. In short, we are standing on the brink of a revolution in cardiovascular care, one based on a more fundamental molecular understanding of disease and the development of new targeted diagnostic strategies and treatments. High-tech approaches such as growing new blood vessels, using stem cells to rebuild diseased organs, and developing artificial organs, long the domain of science fiction, are now real possibilities for future care.

This book, then, weaves together a number of diverse threads. Together, these threads form the fabric of a comprehensive program of cardiovascular health and care. This program involves lifelong maintenance, individualization, patient empowerment, and recognition of the major medical and scientific advances that will form the basis of cardiovascular care for the next decade.

INTRODUCTION

V irtually all heart patients go through a process of trial and error to find a long-term program that fits their lifestyle while providing optimal treatment. They also experience occasional lapses and setbacks. In this book, we describe composite illustrative cases and situations culled from the long-term experience of treating patients. These particular cases highlight issues relating to cardiac care.

Stanley, for example, is a fifty-five-year-old executive whose work requires twelve-hour days and extensive, almost weekly travel. On one of these trips away from home he suffered a small heart attack, and later he had coronary artery bypass surgery. Beyond his hectic work schedule, a number of lifestyle factors worked against his heart health. Perhaps most significantly, he was some fifty pounds overweight. Although he had been an athlete in college, he had long since stopped exercising, citing his arthritic knees and work schedule as excuses. In Chapter 4, you'll learn how he and his doctor worked out a program that allowed him to modify his behavior while still retaining the activities that were important to him and his family.

Alice, a forty-five-year-old part-time school aide, is obese and has type II diabetes, which she treats with oral medication. A routine medical test found high blood cholesterol levels, but rather than take more medication, she elected to try dieting and increasing her exercise. She thought she was making progress until she was suddenly hospitalized after suffering a major heart attack. Her outcome and treatment are described in Chapter 3.

Jennifer's story is very different from Alice's. This trim, healthy-looking fifty-year-old woman has been a long-distance runner since her teenage years, and running is a very important part of her life. She exercises daily, runs one or two marathons a year, and frequently competes in half marathons and 10K events. She had never been aware of any cardiovascular problem, although both parents had heart disease when in their sixties and her brother, only a few years her senior, recently underwent coronary bypass surgery. The first indication that she, too, may have heart disease came after a long run when she developed mild, somewhat atypical, chest discomfort. She finally consulted a doctor when the chest pains become more frequent and intense. Tests showed she had serious coronary artery disease. (Her treatment and long-term program are described in Chapter 2.)

Sam is a fifty-two-year-old school bus driver who smokes two packs of cigarettes a day. He is moderately obese, and does not engage in any physical exercise. His first indication of a possible heart problem came when he developed shortness of breath and a feeling of mild pressure in his chest while walking up a flight of stairs at his home. Because his job involved the safety of dozens of children, his wife insisted that he see a doctor—who diagnosed high blood pressure, mild diabetes, and elevated blood cholesterol and prescribed medications to help with these problems. A more difficult but critical part of Sam's behavior modification program was a requirement that he stop smoking. How he managed to do this and alter other harmful health habits is described in Chapter 5.

John is an eighty-five-year-old retiree who winters in Florida and returns to New England for the spring and summer months. He golfs three times a week, and until recently, generally enjoyed good health. He has longstanding hypertension, which he keeps under control with medication. He also has moderately elevated cholesterol levels, for which he now takes medication. In recent months, he has experienced chest pain whenever he engages in physical activity, even something as moderate as golf. His doctor ordered an exercise stress test, which was markedly abnormal. At Sam's advanced age, should he consider invasive procedures, such as coronary angiography, stenting, or even coronary bypass surgery? (The outcome of his case is described in Chapter 10.)

Although each of these patients likely suffers from the same basic condition of cardiovascular disease, they must be treated as individuals. A forty-five-year-old obese woman with diabetes would be approached quite differently from a fifty-year-old active runner. A program of lifestyle modification for a hard-driving executive must consider his or her business schedule, physical limitations, and overall personality. The approach to symptoms in an individual responsible for driving children to school every day must be far more aggressive than that given to symptoms in an eighty-five-year-old retiree. Still, being eighty-five or even older does not exclude someone as a candidate for surgery or other invasive procedures.

Chapter 1 introduces the concepts of *constants*—the core medical values that doctors use to gauge the nature and severity of disease—and *variables*, the individual characteristics that set you apart from other patients with the same disease. Both must be considered in structuring a lifelong treatment program that works best for you.

The four chapters in Part I deal with lifestyle and heart health; specific topics include exercise, diet, stress and other psychological factors, and smoking. Part II provides a broad overview of the basics of lifelong treatment: diagnostic tests and procedures; medical treatment, surgery, and other interventions; and the role of alternative and complementary therapies.

The six chapters in Part III discuss the needs of different population groups: women, the elderly, minorities, young athletes, adults with congenital heart disease, and travelers with heart disease. The concluding Part IV describes recent advances in and research on promising future therapies; experimental treatments and clinical trials are also discussed.

Throughout this book, you'll find practical advice on how to make small lifestyle changes that can make a big difference in living with cardiovascular disease. You'll also gain insight into the process doctors use in fashioning a long-term program that works best for you. A final word of caution, however: although this book is based on years of experience in treating heart patients as well as the latest scientific advances, you should not use the information to alter your doctor's prescribed regimen. Instead, the information presented here is intended to broaden your understanding of the nature of heart disease, its causes, potential for prevention, and approaches to treatment.

1

A Personalized Plan:
The Key to a Lifelong Heart Program

Although people often think of heart disease as a single, well-defined problem that affects all patients similarly, nothing could be further from reality. Just as no two people are exactly alike, heart disease (and its risk factors, symptoms, and successful treatments) varies greatly from one person to another. In our experience, a one-plan-fits-all approach—be it diet, medication, or lifestyle modification—simply does not work. Thus, an essential first step toward developing your lifelong heart health regimen is to identify what makes you different from your parents, siblings, neighbors, and the other patients in your doctor's office. This is why the concept of *constants* and *individual variables* is so important.

Many scientific studies have identified the constants, the core medical values that guide physicians in the diagnosis of cardiovascular disease. Large population studies, such as the Framingham Heart Study, pinpoint the risk factors doctors look for in identifying patients who may have or are likely to develop heart disease. The Framingham study, an ongoing exhaustive research project, was started in 1948 and over the decades has followed the health status of thousands of residents of Framingham, Massachusetts, over several generations. As a result of such studies, doctors now have solid evidence linking a number of lifestyle, hereditary, and health factors to an increased risk of a heart attack. The Framingham study also demonstrates that eliminating or modifying these risk factors reduces the likelihood of a heart attack. For example, your doctor should always check your cholesterol levels. This is a constant. But he must also account for your variability. Can elevated levels be treated with diet or is medicine necessary? Which medicine? How often should it be checked? What happens as you get older? What happens if you exercise more? The same applies to high blood pressure and the other major risk factors.

Such large-scale population studies form the basis of much of our current medical knowledge. But there are always exceptions; we all have known or heard about individuals who smoke three packs a day, never exercise, eat fat-laden red meat every day, ignore doctors' advice (if they even go to a doctor at all), and still live long lives. Clearly, such people defy the odds. Yet playing such odds is a very risky business. A much wiser approach involves optimizing your chances for a healthful future by defining your personal risk profile (constants or core medical values) and then working with your doctor to define your individual variables and devise a long-term plan to minimize risk. This makes your lifelong treatment or preventive program different from other seemingly similar individuals. And this is where your individual variables come into play.

Some risk factors—your age, blood pressure, cholesterol, and so forth—are obvious or easily identified. Others are more subtle yet may be equally fundamental in determining the long-term success of your treatment. Only you can home in on many of these individual variables. What is your mindset? Are you in a state of denial, ignoring clear warning signs? In contrast, do you (or your spouse) obsess over every little twinge? Helping you answer such questions is a focus of this book.

In this chapter, we first describe the various cardiovascular risk factors (the constants) and briefly outline some of the more common variables that doctors should consider in working with you to develop a realistic and effective management program. We also list common warning signs and symptoms, again taking into consideration important individual variables. Finally, we offer guidelines for finding a doctor who will become your partner in managing your health care.

Let's start by considering the risk factors that increase your chances of developing some form of heart or blood vessel disease. The fewer of these you have, the lower your chances of developing heart disease. Similarly, your chances are improved by reducing or eliminating as many risk factors as possible.

INBORN OR GENETIC RISK FACTORS

First, let's consider those risk factors that are beyond your control. Remember, however, that even if you have one or more of these risk factors, you need not sit back and await your fate. First of all, the differences between your genes and those of family members can change the odds. And even though you can't change inborn risk factors, there is a good deal you can do to modulate their presumed effects. Within each of the following categories are many variables that you can alter as part of your individualized treatment and preventive program.

Age

Although it would be a huge mistake to assume you're somehow immune to heart disease because you're still in your thirties, forties, or fifties, it is clear that cardiovascular risk rises with advancing age. More than half of all heart attacks occur in persons over the age of sixty-five, and 80 percent of those who die of heart disease are in this age bracket. But given that cardiovascular disease claims as many as a million people each year, a huge number of younger people are also at risk.

Obviously, you can't turn back or stop the clock, but lifestyle factors—such as diet, exercise, and stress management—certainly minimize the adverse effects of advancing age. How you modify your lifestyle also varies greatly depending on your age. For example, exercise is important at any age, but a regimen that works well for a forty-year-old may be difficult or impossible for an eighty-year-old to maintain. Cholesterol levels and blood pressure rise naturally with increasing age, so what's dangerous for a thirty-year-old may well be acceptable for an eighty-five-year-old and not require treatment. This is a controversial area. In contrast, systolic blood pressure—the first (higher) of the two numbers in a blood-pressure reading—often rises to unacceptably high levels in older people, even though the diastolic pressure (the second, or lower, number) may be normal. This type of systolic hypertension requires treatment to reduce the risk of a heart attack or stroke (see Chapter 7).

Symptoms also can vary with age; for example, irregular heartbeats that are benign in a young person may signal a serious problem in someone who is older. In addition, older people are more likely to have other diseases that increase the risk or compound the effects of heart disease.

Age also affects which treatments will work best. Medications that work well in a young person, for example, may be inappropriate or prescribed in a different dosage for someone a few decades older. (See Chapter 10 for a more detailed discussion of older patients' specific needs.)

Gender

Heart disease is by far the leading cause of death in both men and women, but there are important gender differences in risk, diagnosis, and treatment. The reasons for these differences are not fully understood, although anatomy and hormones undoubtedly play important roles. For example, women have smaller coronary arteries than men—a consideration when treating coronary artery disease. In addition, women with heart disease often experience symptoms different from those of their male counterparts. When a woman has a heart attack, she may experience little or no pain, and when pain occurs, it may be centered more in the back and abdomen than in the mid-chest. As a result, many women delay seeking medical attention or assume the problem is indigestion or a backache rather than a heart attack. In contrast, men are more likely to experience crushing or severe chest pain, which leaves little doubt that something is wrong with the heart.

Women face an increasing risk of a heart attack after menopause, when estrogen production falls dramatically. Until the last few years, doctors attributed the increased risk to a lack of estrogen and many prescribed hormone replacement therapy (HRT) as a preventive measure. But we now know that estrogen alone is not the whole story. A 2004 report by the Women's Health Initiative Study, a long-term research project coordinated by the National Institutes of Health, showed that estrogen replacement after menopause may actually raise the risk of a heart attack or stroke. This finding differed from earlier studies, including the 1989 report on the Nurses' Health Study (see Chapter 9 for a more detailed discussion).

Heart disease tends to develop at a younger age in men than women, and men are more vulnerable to sudden cardiac death. But after menopause, women begin to "catch up" with men, and overall, more women than men die of heart disease each year. Still, many people—both doctors and patients—mistakenly think that women are somehow immune to heart disease and tend to discount early warning signs and symptoms until a woman's condition reaches an advanced stage. All too many women still mistakenly think that breast cancer is their number one health risk. In reality, the risk of suffering a fatal heart attack is many times higher than that of succumbing to breast cancer. Obviously, this does not mean that women should ignore the risk of breast cancer. But periodic assessment of cardiovascular risk is just as important for a woman as getting a mammogram every year or two.

Family History

We've known for many decades that people with a strong family history of heart attacks, stroke, and other cardiovascular disorders face an increased risk of suffering similar fates. This has been amply demonstrated by the Framingham Heart Study and other large population studies. The risk is highest among those whose close relatives (sibling, parent, or grandparent) suffered a heart attack before age fifty.

There are also genetic disorders that increase cardiovascular risk. For example, some people inherit a gene that results in very high levels of LDL cholesterol, the bad form of this blood lipid, leading to early coronary artery disease. Some forms of heart muscle disease also run in families. Although you can't change your genetic makeup, there are many preventive steps you can take to escape the fate of your forebears. Start by discussing your family history with your doctor, who may want to do specific diagnostic tests to detect silent heart disease. With the help of your doctor, you can then adopt a lifelong prevention or treatment program.

Race and Ethnic Background

Certain racial or ethnic groups have an especially high risk of heart disease. At highest risk are African Americans, Mexican Americans, Native Americans, native Hawaiians, and people from the Indian subcontinent. We are only beginning to understand some of the genetic factors that increase vulnerability. For example, African Americans tend to be highly salt-sensitive, which increases their risk of high blood pressure. Mexican Americans tend to have more hypertension than other Latino groups, which may explain their increased vulnerability. Some Native Americans have a very high incidence of diabetes, which also increases their cardiovascular risk. Other factors that may play a role include unidentified genetic differences, diet, stress, low income, and limited access to health care. Again, early intervention and extra attention to a heart-healthy lifestyle can go a long way toward dealing with these risk factors in all populations. (See Chapter 11 for a more detailed discussion.)

ACQUIRED RISK FACTORS

The list of acquired risk factors, which can be changed or prevented, is much longer than those that are beyond our control. Reducing or eliminating these risk factors is key to achieving and maintaining heart health, so they deserve special attention.

Elevated Blood Cholesterol and Other Lipids

Cholesterol is a fatty substance (lipid) that circulates in the blood and is essential to maintaining life. Indeed, every cell in the body must have a certain amount of cholesterol in order to function properly. The body can make all of the cholesterol it needs; it is also found in all animal products, especially eggs, whole milk, and fatty meats. Thus, a diet high in such foods can raise blood cholesterol levels. In addition, foods that include tropical oils (palm, palm kernel, and coconut oils) and transfatty acids (fats that have been artificially hardened) raise cholesterol, and reducing intake of these foods can help lower elevated cholesterol.

Cholesterol becomes a problem when too much circulates in the blood. This may be due to diet, or to the tendency for cholesterol to rise with age, but sometimes the body simply makes too much cholesterol, perhaps due to genetic differences. Regardless of the underlying cause, high blood cholesterol can lead to atherosclerosis, the buildup of fatty deposits (plaque) in the coronary arteries and other blood vessels. But the story is more complicated than simply having too much cholesterol circulating in the blood. Because cholesterol and other lipids are fats and blood is mostly water (and fats and water don't mix), in order for cholesterol to circulate in the blood it must be attached to water-soluble substances. These are proteins, which when combined with cholesterol are called lipoproteins. The type of lipoprotein is a key factor in determining the degree of potential harm from high cholesterol. Low-density lipoproteins, or LDL cholesterol, form the so-called "bad" cholesterol. This is because high LDL levels can form fatty deposits in the arteries. In time, this plaque can narrow the coronary arteries, setting the stage for coronary artery disease and a heart attack.

In contrast, high-density lipoprotein, or HDL cholesterol—the so-called "good" cholesterol—prevents the buildup of fatty plaque by carrying lipids away from the artery walls and returning it to the liver to be reprocessed or eliminated from the body. In general, experts agree the ratio of HDL to LDL cholesterol is a prime predictor of coronary artery disease, heart attack, and stroke. But how high or low each should be is still open to debate. It has long been accepted that a total cholesterol of less than 200 mg/dl (milligrams per deciliter) should be the goal for most people. More important, however, is the level of LDL cholesterol, which should be below 100 mg/dl in people free of heart disease and 80 mg/dl or less in people who have been diagnosed as having coronary artery disease. In addition, the higher the levels of HDL cholesterol, the better. At a minimum, your HDL should be 40 mg/dl.

In determining the best approach to lowering high blood cholesterol, a doctor will look at a number of variables: diet, weight, exercise habits, genetics, the existence of diabetes and other diseases, age, and gender, among others. For people with high LDL cholesterol, drugs called statins are especially beneficial because they lower LDL cholesterol while promoting a higher level of the protective HDL cholesterol. Elevated triglycerides, another lipid that is a factor in increased cardiovascular risk, can usually be controlled by diet and possibly exercise. If these measures are inadequate, other medication may be prescribed. (See Chapter 7 for a more in-depth discussion.)

High Blood Pressure

Often called the silent killer, high blood pressure (or "hypertension") produces no obvious symptoms until it reaches the advanced stage and damages organs, especially the kidneys, heart, brain, and blood vessels. It is one of the most common risk factors for heart attack, stroke, kidney failure, peripheral vascular disease, atherosclerosis, and heart failure, defined as an inability of the heart to pump enough blood to meet the body's needs. Untreated, it can also lead to left ventricular hypertrophy (LVH), an enlargement and thickening of the walls of the heart's main pumping chamber. LVH is an independent risk factor for heart failure.

In general, high blood pressure is defined as consistent blood pressure readings above 140/90, although 120/80 is the goal. Although hypertension is bad for everyone, African Americans are especially vulnerable to developing it and to suffering its complications. Reasons for this include the increased salt sensitivity and greater incidence of obesity and diabetes in this population group. Regardless of the underlying cause, when compared to other racial and ethnic populations, African Americans are more likely to suffer severe consequences from high blood pressure, including kidney failure, congestive heart failure, and stroke.

Women also have an increased risk of developing high blood pressure, especially if they are overweight, have a family history of the disease, or are over the age of fifty. Some studies have found that nearly three out of four American women over the age of sixty-five have high blood pressure. Fortunately, most high blood pressure can be controlled with a combination of lifestyle factors (diet, exercise, weight control) and antihypertensive medication. (See Chapter 7 for treatment guidelines.)

Metabolic Syndrome

Metabolic syndrome is a constellation of risk factors that tend to occur together. Although it is very common, affecting more than 40 percent of Americans over age sixty, it has only recently been defined as a major cardiovascular risk factor. Diagnosis is based on a patient's having three or more of the following risk factors: abdominal obesity (a waist circumference greater than forty inches in a man and thirty-five inches in a woman), elevated triglycerides (a blood level of 150 mg/dl or higher), low HDL cholesterol (blood levels lower than 40 mg/dl in men and 50 mg/dl in women), high blood pressure (more than 130/85), and insulin resistance (defined as a fasting blood sugar of 100 mg/dl or higher along with elevated insulin levels).

Metabolic syndrome poses a double risk because it not only increases your chances of developing cardiovascular disease but is also strongly linked to the development of type II diabetes. Consequently, doctors now pay more attention to the syndrome when developing a treatment program. For example, moderately elevated cholesterol may be treated more vigorously in a person with other components of metabolic syndrome than in someone without them. In addition to treating individual components of the syndrome, doctors work with patients to institute lifestyle changes to halt progression to heart disease and/or diabetes. Important variables that should be considered include weight, age, racial and ethnic background, and the status of any of the individual components of metabolic syndrome.

Diabetes and Insulin Resistance

There is no doubt that persons with diabetes mellitus, both type I and type II, have an increased risk of heart attacks, stroke, and other cardiovascular diseases. Even persons who do not have established diabetes but have slightly elevated levels of blood sugar and circulating insulin—the hormone that maintains normal blood sugar—are at increased risk. The risk is further increased in persons with metabolic syndrome, in which other risk factors are present (see earlier). This accumulation of risk is increasingly worrisome given the current epidemic of obesity and a skyrocketing incidence of type II, or insulin-resistant, diabetes among young adults and even teenagers.

A significant percentage of type II diabetes can be controlled or prevented by diet and exercise, but many studies have found that very few people stick to their recommended regimens. This is why it's important to work with your doctor to develop an individualized diet and exercise program that takes into consideration your preferences. Doctors are also increasingly turning to diabetes medications to treat type II diabetes. If your doctor recommends such medications as part of your treatment, you will need to work together to find the drug that controls blood sugar without causing serious side effects.

Obesity

Until recently, most people considered being overweight more a matter of aesthetics than a potentially deadly disease. Then came a rash of studies in the 1980s and 1990s identifying excess weight as a major health risk, and proposing that the greater the weight, the higher the risk of developing heart disease, hypertension, diabetes, and other serious health problems. Obesity—defined as a body-mass index (BMI) of 30 or higher—is now accepted as a leading cause of premature death. But the same may not apply to modest overweight, a BMI of 25 to 29.9. A 2005 report from the Centers for Disease Control found that people whose weight fell in this range actually had a lower risk of premature death than people who were markedly underweight—a BMI of less than 18.4. (To determine your BMI, consult Table 2 in Chapter 3.)

Still, there is no doubt that obesity increases the risk for heart disease and needs treatment. Doctors now recognize that obesity is a disease, and not just a matter of weak willpower or a desire for sugary, fatty foods (although these are certainly contributing factors). Indeed, researchers are just beginning to home in on the root causes of obesity, which may include genetics, metabolism, hormonal factors, and as yet unidentified factors.

Even though the causes of obesity are not fully understood, it can be prevented or treated. But as with other acquired risk factors, there are many variables that must be considered. For example, the distribution of body fat is an important factor in determining its risk. Fat is metabolically active, and the distribution of excessive fat determines its level of danger. Apple-shaped persons with a large beer belly, or android or truncal obesity, are more likely to have high blood cholesterol, low HDL cholesterol, diabetes, and high blood pressure than the so-called pear-shaped persons, whose fat is more evenly distributed or concentrated in the thighs and buttocks. This is because abdominal fat is more metabolically active than fats stored in other parts of the body. Younger men are more susceptible than women to developing android obesity, but this changes following menopause, when women, too, tend to accumulate more abdominal fat. Other variables include age, the ability (or motivation) to exercise, education, and socioeconomic factors. Ethnicity and customs may also play a role. For example, many people of African or Hispanic origin consider obesity physically attractive and a sign of prosperity and even good health, whereas persons of European origin regard excessive weight as physically unattractive and a sign of weak willpower.

Cigarette Smoking

Cigarette use is now recognized as the single most common cause of premature death in the United States and many other countries. Although most people know that smoking increases the risk of many forms of cancer, many are unaware of its role in cardiovascular disease, including sudden cardiac death, heart attacks, and strokes. Smoking also increases the risk of congestive heart failure and circulatory disorders. Smokers who have a heart attack are much more likely to die than nonsmokers, even though they tend to be thinner and have fewer other risk factors. Even secondhand smoke increases risk.

The good news is that quitting smoking reduces the risk of premature death from heart disease. According to the American Heart Association, a person's risk is cut in half within a year of stopping smoking and in time, it is about the same as that of nonsmokers. But as most smokers can testify, quitting can be very difficult because nicotine, the active ingredient in tobacco products, is highly addictive.

Tobacco use involves a number of variables, including education, age, family influences, stress, and peer pressure, and these are important considerations for determining not only who starts smoking but also who will have the most difficult time quitting. Although there are many exceptions, in general college-educated people are less likely to smoke than people with less education. In addition, many studies have found that the longer people go without smoking, the less likely they are to start. For example, most smokers begin when they are in their early teens, whereas very few people take up smoking when they are in their twenties or thirties. Children whose parents smoke are also more likely to smoke than children of nonsmokers. Peer pressure is often cited as the number one reason youngsters start smoking; adolescents universally want to be "one of the gang," and all too many mistakenly think smoking makes them appear cool.

Gender also plays a role. Women tend to have more difficulty quitting than men, even though the consequences of continued smoking may be more serious for women than men. For women smokers, like all smokers, analyzing the motives for tobacco use can be helpful for finding the best way to quit. For example, many young women take up smoking because they think it will prevent weight gain, and they often resist quitting because of fears of getting fat. For these women, combining smoking cessation with a diet and exercise program to prevent weight gain can be very helpful. (See Chapter 5 for more specific suggestions on how to beat cigarette addiction.)

Stress

Doctors have long debated the role of stress in promoting heart disease, but there's a growing body of evidence that it is a risk factor. Exactly how stress harms the heart is not fully understood, but researchers do know that constant high levels of stress prompt hormonal changes that can send blood pressure and insulin levels soaring, and likely promote inflammation and other body changes that, over time, increase cardiovascular risk. Stress may also lead to depression, one of several psychological factors linked to an increased risk of a heart attack.

Both short-term and prolonged stress appear to be risk factors. Many heart attack patients report undergoing unusual stress in the hours before they were stricken. It is well-known that sudden, severe stress can precipitate a heart attack in people who already have coronary disease. For example, heart attack deaths rose sharply in the days immediately after the 1994 Northridge earthquake in Los Angeles and during the Scud missile attacks on Israel during the first Gulf war.

Sustained stress has also been associated with an increased heart-attack risk. This connection was documented in a recent multinational study that surveyed more than eleven thousand people who had suffered heart attacks and compared them with about thirteen thousand healthy control subjects. The study found that the heart-attack patients had been under much more stress in the previous year than had been the healthy controls. The stress came from various sources—problems at work, financial difficulties, family troubles, depression, the death of a loved one, and other causes. The senior investigator of the study, Dr. Salim Yusuf of McMaster University, concluded that stress "was comparable to risk factors like hypertension and abdominal obesity," and that its effect was "much greater than we thought before."

Of course, all of us are subjected to different types of stress every day, and most people can develop moderately effective ways of dealing with it. Yet the presence of other risk factors and a person's personality make everyone's experience of stress unique. A hard-driven executive may thrive on a stress level that would drive other people crazy. Conversely, even low levels of stress may tip the balance for a more high-strung person. In any event, persistent stress and poor coping mechanisms can harm health. (See Chapter 4 for helpful ways to manage stress.)

Other Psychological Factors

Several studies published in the last few years have identified depression as an independent factor that increases the risk of a heart attack. Precisely how depression affects heart function is unknown, but diagnosing and treating depression is now considered an important aspect of reducing cardiovascular risk. (See Chapter 4.)

Sedentary Lifestyle

Numerous studies have found that exercise is an important factor in preventing or treating heart disease. People who exercise regularly not only live longer than their sedentary counterparts, but they also feel and look better. They are less likely to be overweight and develop other cardiovascular risk factors, including diabetes, high blood pressure, and elevated blood cholesterol. But even though most people know that regular exercise is beneficial, many have difficulty sticking to a regimen. Arthritis and other orthopedic problems, weight, weather, geographic locale, time constraints, and availability of exercise facilities are just some of the obstacles to a successful exercise program. Indeed, we all can probably come up with a long list of excuses to remain a sedentary "couch potato," but in fact virtually everyone can develop an exercise program that fits his or her lifestyle. If you have arthritic knees, jogging or singles tennis is not going to be part of your long-term exercise regimen. But you may well consider swimming, tai chi, using an elliptical trainer, or any number of other enjoyable activities. (See Chapter 2 for more ideas.)

NEWLY IDENTIFIED RISK FACTORS

Our understanding of the causes and treatments of heart disease is expanding daily. So it is not surprising that from time to time, new risk factors are identi-

fied. Not enough is known about these risk factors to pinpoint common variables, but doctors are increasingly considering the following variables in assessing a patient's total health picture.

Fibrinogen

Fibrinogen is a component of blood that promotes the formation of blood clots.
Although it is essential for stopping bleeding from cuts and other wounds, high
levels raise the risk of a heart attack—or a stroke if a clot were to block the essential flow of blood to the heart or brain. Fibrinogen levels tend to rise with advancing age; smoking also promotes increased fibrinogen production. Many experts believe this is one reason why smoking greatly increases cardiovascular risk.

Lipoprotein (a)

Often abbreviated as Lp(a), Lipoprotein (a) was discovered in 1963, and a number of studies in the last decade link it to an increased risk of coronary artery disease and heart attacks. Lp(a) is the component of LDL (the carrier of the harmful
type of cholesterol) that prevents blood clots from dissolving normally. Studies
have shown that high levels of Lp(a) are perhaps more important in predicting the
likelihood of a heart attack than is high total cholesterol or low HDL cholesterol.
Increasingly, then, doctors are measuring Lp(a) levels to try to better understand
the relationship among these variables and more effectively advise their patients.
Lowering LDL cholesterol may help reduce levels of Lp(a), and researchers are
studying the possible role of high doses of nicotinic acid (one of the B vitamins)
to specifically lower it.

Inflammation and C-reactive Protein

Over the past decade, doctors have paid increasing attention to the possible link
between chronic inflammation and heart disease. Indeed, some studies indicate
that high levels of C-reactive protein, or CRP, may be a risk factor even when a
patient's cholesterol is normal, because CRP is a protein in the blood that indicates inflammation somewhere in the body, and because chronic inflammatory
disorders such as rheumatoid arthritis have been associated with an increased
risk of heart disease. The precise mechanism is unknown, but some have theorized that an underlying bacterial or viral infection may contribute to, or even
cause, the buildup of fatty plaque along arterial walls. Regardless of the cause, in-

flammation in the arteries appears to promote the development of atherosclerosis and instability of the atherosclerotic plaque that can lead to formation of blood clots, which can further block blood flow and result in a heart attack or stroke.

A great deal of research has gone on over the past five years defining the role of CRP as a risk factor. Normally there are very low levels (1.0 mg/L or less) of CRP in the blood. Levels are readily measured by a simple blood test, referred to as hs-CRP (for "high-sensitivity CRP"), which is now widely available. An hs-CRP test may be especially important in pinpointing persons at very high risk of a heart attack or stroke. The test predicts elevated risk regardless of gender or age, and is most important for persons who are already at high risk of having a heart attack. For example, a high CRP level points to a very high risk of a heart attack in patients with unstable angina (chest pain that occurs during rest) or those who have had a previous heart attack. Recent studies indicate that high hs-CRP (3.0 mg/L or more) is a more powerful predictor of a heart attack, sudden cardiac death, and stroke than are high cholesterol and certain other risk factors. In any event, we now recommend that anyone with a high risk of cardiovascular disease receive hs-CRP testing, and if this is elevated, undergo intensive preventive treatment. In the future this may become a routine screening test.

Homocysteine

Homocysteine is an amino acid that is a natural part of protein metabolism. Some people inherit a genetic defect that causes them to produce very high levels of homocysteine, putting them at a high risk of developing severe atherosclerosis and suffering an early heart attack. In addition, many people have elevated homocysteine levels without the inherited genetic disorder and they, too, have an elevated heart-disease risk. So in addition to measuring cholesterol and other blood components, many doctors now routinely test for elevated homocysteine. It is easily reduced with large doses of folic acid; in some instances, other B vitamins are added to the regimen.

Sleep Apnea

When a person stops breathing during brief periods while sleeping, he or she is said to have sleep apnea. Many people with sleep apnea are unaware of the disorder, but their bed partners can describe what happens. Typically, the sufferer—most often an overweight middle-aged man—thrashes about restlessly during sleep, with loud snoring interrupted by moments of silence during which there is no noticeable breathing. At this point the person partially wakes with a start, then resumes a fitful sleep. Because sleep can be interrupted by many episodes of half waking, the person feels abnormally drowsy during the day.

People with sleep apnea have an increased risk of sudden cardiac death while sleeping. Preventive approaches include losing weight and perhaps using a breathing device that helps regulate respiration during sleep. Removal of the tonsils and adenoids helps some people, and in extreme cases, other types of surgery may be considered.

Cocaine Use

Every now and then, the sudden death of a seemingly healthy young athlete makes headlines. All too often, these deaths are linked to cocaine use. Unfortunately, the risk is not limited to athletes; escalating cocaine use has led to an increase in high blood pressure, abnormal heart rhythms, angina, cardiomyopathy (a disease of the heart muscle), and heart attacks among young people. Cocaine use during pregnancy also increases the risk of congenital heart defects.

Even the first use of cocaine can lead to a cardiac crisis, heart attack, and even death. This is because cocaine has a number of almost immediate adverse effects on the heart. It reduces blood flow to the heart muscle by constricting the coronary arteries, which can result in a coronary artery spasm. At the same time, it speeds up the heart rate and increases blood pressure. As a result, the amount of oxygen reaching the heart muscle itself is reduced just when the heart muscle is demanding more oxygen.

RECOGNIZING SIGNS AND SYMPTOMS OF HEART DISEASE

Of all people with heart disease, half or more go undiagnosed until the disease reaches an advanced stage. Tragically, a heart attack or even sudden death is the initial sign or symptom in all too many instances. Early diagnosis and treatment are absolutely essential. But who should be screened for possible heart disease? Obviously, people with a number of the risk factors discussed on previous pages should be especially alert for possible symptoms. But even low-risk, seemingly healthy persons can have high blood pressure, clogged coronary arteries, and other silent forms of cardiovascular disease. Many of these disorders can be detected by a routine medical checkup, something we recommend every year or two for everyone over the age of forty and for younger persons with a number of risk factors.

Just as risk factors differ greatly from one person to another, so do symptoms. In evaluating a patient, doctors take into consideration many factors in addition to the obvious symptoms. These include biological and sociological factors, including age, gender, ethnic background, communication skills, and self-image.

Sometimes there are no obvious warning symptoms until a heart attack occurs. Even in these cases, however, it is often learned later that important warning symptoms were ignored. Some patients, for example, experience for several months shortness of breath and chest discomfort during exercise, but wait until the symptoms become very severe or occur during rest before seeking medical help. At the opposite extreme, every day emergency room physicians see people who are convinced they are having a heart attack when in reality the problem is a panic attack, heartburn, spasm of the esophagus, or another benign condition. The trick is to strike a balance between denial and hypersensitivity.

Textbooks list a number of classic signs and symptoms of heart disease, but it is important to stress that there are many individual combinations and variations. One or more of the following symptoms may occur, but you may also experience other warning signs of heart disease not listed here. Be sure to consult your physician if you have a serious concern about your symptoms.

Chest Pain

Pain in the chest is the most worrisome symptom of heart disease and should never be ignored. Still, not all chest pain signals heart disease, just as not every headache stems from a brain tumor. Thus, our first task is to determine the cause of the pain (see Box 1). As a general rule, any unusual or unprovoked chest pain that lasts more than two minutes needs to be checked by a doctor as soon as possible. All too often people experiencing a heart attack wait hours before seeking medical attention, and by then it may be too late. As noted, this does not mean that every twinge requires a trip to the emergency room. The very nature of the chest pain provides important clues. Is it a constant, squeezing pain that lasts more than two minutes? Does it radiate to the arm(s), back, neck, or jaw? Is it provoked by exercise, exposure to the cold, or emotional stress? Is it occurring with increasing frequency? A yes answer to any of these questions warrants an immediate call to your doctor or for emergency medical services. An electrocardiogram (ECG) and perhaps an exercise stress test can help determine whether the pain arises in the heart. Chest pain that disappears after taking nitroglycerine also points to a possible heart problem, although this drug will also ease an esophageal spasm.

Box 1

POSSIBLE CAUSES OF CHEST PAIN

- Coronary artery disease (angina pectoris)
- Heart attack or acute coronary syndrome (ACS)
- Heartburn (gastric reflux) or inflammation of the esophagus
- Hiatal hernia
- Gallbladder disease
- Peptic ulcer
- Musculoskeletal disorders
- Mitral valve prolapse
- Aortic aneurysm
- Pericarditis (inflammation of the membrane surrounding the heart)
- Lung disorders such as pneumonia, a collapsed lung (pneumothorax), or a pulmonary embolism
- Panic attacks and other anxiety disorders

Shortness of Breath

Shortness of breath, or dyspnea, is one of the most common early symptoms of cardiovascular problems, but it can have many other causes. So your doctor will ask a number of questions when trying to determine whether it is related to heart function. Does it come on only after heavy exertion? If so, the shortness of breath may be natural or indicate you're out of shape. Do you experience shortness of breath when you're under emotional stress? In this case, your symptom may be a manifestation of anxiety. In contrast, do you experience shortness of breath when engaging in normal activities, such as moderate walking or even when you're resting? Does it come on suddenly? Does it waken you at night? Do you often feel like you cannot get enough air into your lungs, even when breathing deeply? See a doctor as soon as possible if the answer to any of these last four questions is yes.

Palpitations or Irregular Heartbeats

The heart ordinarily beats in a steady rhythm, slowing down when we are resting or asleep and speeding up when we exercise or are under stress. Most of the time we are not aware of our heartbeat, even when it speeds up or slows down. But you may be very aware of palpitations or a cardiac arrhythmia. Sometimes the causes are self-evident or easily diagnosed. For example, do the palpitations come on after drinking several cups of coffee or indulging in alcohol? If so, try cutting back and see if they go away. Did you first notice the problem after starting a new medication? If so, ask your doctor if the irregular heartbeat is due to an adverse drug reaction. Do you experience the palpitation during periods of heavy stress? If so, try meditation or another calming technique. Persistent irregular heartbeats, however, should be investigated.

Most palpitations are more of a nuisance than a serious medical condition. But more serious disorders such as an abnormality in the heart's electrical activity should be ruled out. To help identify the underlying cause, your doctor will ask you to describe the irregularities. For example, when does the irregular heartbeat occur? If you are aware of it mostly at night or when you are alone, it may simply indicate you are more conscious of a minor irregularity when you are not distracted by daily activities. Does the sensation feel like a fluttering or pounding in the chest? Does the heart seem to be skipping beats or flip-flopping? Are the palpitations accompanied by feelings of dizziness or even fainting? Irregular heartbeats can sometimes be diagnosed by listening to the heart and doing an ECG. But more often, the irregularities are intermittent and may not occur while you're in a doctor's office. In such cases, doctors can use a Holter monitor, a portable device that takes a continuous ECG over twenty-four or forty-eight hours or perhaps even longer.

Fainting Spells

Fainting spells, or syncope, typically occur when the brain is deprived of oxygen for more than a few seconds. Fainting has many causes (see Box 2), but one of the more common causes involves an abnormal response of the vagus nerve. This nerve controls many functions, including blood flow to the abdomen. During a vasovagal episode, the heartbeat slows, blood pressure drops, and blood flow to the brain is reduced, which leads to dizziness and fainting. A vasovagal response can be prompted by many experiences, including pain, the sight of blood, dehydration, odors, and fright. Other types of interactions between the nervous system and the heart can also produce "neurocardiogenic syncope," which may occur in response to other conditions such as prolonged standing or intense exercise. More serious are heart-related causes of fainting. These include abnormal heart rhythms, such as a very slow or very rapid heartbeat. In general, a fainting episode—especially recurrent spells—warrants medical investigation to rule out serious causes.

Swelling or Puffiness

Fluid retention around the ankles and legs (edema), in the abdomen (ascites), or in the lungs often signals a heart problem, such as an inability to pump blood adequately. The nature of the swelling may point to a likely cause. For example, swelling of the ankles and lower legs can be caused by pumping failure of the right side of the heart. (Such swelling can also be due to abnormalities of the venous system, such as varicose veins, or simply a lack of exercise.) Abdominal edema and leg swelling may also signal right-sided heart failure. In contrast, fluid in the lungs is often due to left-sided heart failure.

Before assuming that edema is a sign of heart failure, however, a doctor must rule out other possible causes. These include kidney disorders, diseases of the veins (venous insufficiency), liver disease, allergies, or a reaction to certain drugs, especially certain calcium channel blockers used to treat high blood pressure or angina pectoris.

Persistent Fatigue

Fatigue is a very common, highly subjective symptom with many causes, including heart disease. Although almost any disease can cause fatigue, the nature of the tiredness often indicates its cause. For example, do you wake up feeling energetic but then suffer fatigue that builds up during the day? Is it accompanied by a feeling of heaviness or weakness of the legs? Is there also shortness of breath? If so, the fatigue may be caused by an inability of the heart to pump enough blood. But before concluding that the heart is the problem, doctors must rule out a number of other diseases as well as sleep disorders and psychological causes such as depression.

Again, few heart patients exhibit classic textbook symptoms: in fact, a quarter or more of all heart attacks are "silent" and are detected only later, typically during a routine ECG. A doctor establishing a diagnosis of heart disease must take into account a number of factors, including gender, age, and life circumstances, among others. For example, women often do not experience typical chest pain or angina; instead, they may complain of fatigue, vague backaches, indigestion, or a feeling of unease—symptoms that are often dismissed as psychologi-

Box 2

CAUSES OF FAINTING

- Slow heartbeat
- Cardiac arrhythmias, including a very fast heartbeat
- Low blood pressure
- Sinus node dysfunction (a disorder of the heart's electrical system)
- Vasovagal episode
- Neurocardiogenic dysfunction
- Narrowing of the neck's carotid artery, which carries blood to the brain
- Narrowing (stenosis) of the aortic valve
- Low blood sugar (hypoglycemia)
- Adverse drug reaction, especially to medications used for treating high blood pressure
- Epilepsy
- Severe anemia or blood loss

cal rather than physical. An older person troubled by difficulty sleeping may assume that age rather than congestive heart failure is the cause. A hard-driving executive may ignore symptoms or attribute them to stress. In contrast, an anxious or worried individual may assume any minor twinge or bout of indigestion foretells an impending heart attack. Striking a balance between denial and unwarranted concern is the key to appropriate surveillance and action.

CHOOSING A DOCTOR

Until now, we have concentrated on your characteristics as a patient. The next step is to develop a partnership with a doctor who's right for you. Many people find this one of the most challenging hurdles in developing and following a long-term health regimen. Just as no two patients are alike, doctors also have different attitudes and approaches, and it is important to find one who meets your needs and expectations. Obviously medical skills and training are important, but so too are attitude, empathy, the ability to listen, and communication skills. For you and your doctor to enter into a long-term relationship, the two of you should fashion a workable plan that not only takes into account your symptoms and risk factors, but also considers your lifestyle, age, gender, economic situation, and myriad other individual variables.

We advise starting the process by listing the questions important to you. Some possibilities are listed here:

Is now the right time? All too often, people put off seeing a doctor for any number of reasons: "I thought the symptoms would go away on their own." "I've got too many other things going on to take the time to find a doctor." "I'm getting older and what good is it going to do to see a doctor now?" No doubt you can add a number of other excuses. Still, if you have unexplained or troubling symptoms, you should see a doctor, and the sooner the better. If you are developing a heart problem, delay only allows it to worsen, whereas early intervention may well halt or even reverse the process.

Who is the right doctor? In general, the best place to start is with a primary-care physician—typically an internist or family physician who has broad training in general medicine. (Many women look to an obstetrician/gynecologist for their primary care, but this medical specialist is not the best choice for dealing with potential heart problems.) There are exceptions, however. Starting with a cardiologist may be the best first choice if you are at high risk of a heart attack and are experiencing chest pains, shortness of breath, or other potentially heart-related symptoms.

How do I find the right doctor? Unfortunately, there is no easy answer to this question, especially given today's fragmented medical system. If you are in a health maintenance organization or similar program, you must start by reviewing the plan's list of medical providers. You might talk to others in the plan for advice concerning practitioners. If you are able to select a doctor outside of your medical plan, ask friends or family members for recommendations. Names can also be gathered by calling a local medical society or teaching hospital, or checking the web sites of professional societies such as the American College of Cardiology. There are also online referral sites, but use caution when consulting these; some are simply personal advertisements, whereas others sponsored by medical centers or hospitals may be more reliable.

When you have a list of names, you can consult library reference books such as the American Medical Association's *Directory of Medical Specialists*. These sources provide an overview of a doctor's education, training, certification, general age, and other background facts. Ask yourself what you feel is important in a doctor. Are you more comfortable with a male or female physician? Do you prefer an older, more experienced doctor—or would you rather work with someone who is younger?

The next step involves calling the doctors' offices to ask a few preliminary questions: Is the doctor taking new patients? Does he or she accept your insurance? What is the charge for a routine office visit? What is his or her hospital affiliation? (You should have confidence in the hospital at which you would receive in-patient treatment.) Is he or she in a solo or group practice, and if a solo practitioner, who assists the patients when the doctor is away?

After you have identified a list of prospective doctors, try to set up a first visit. In only a few minutes, you should be able to tell if the doctor will be a suitable partner in your long-term care. Questions to ask yourself include: Does he or she listen patiently and thoughtfully to what I'm saying? Is this doctor willing to answer questions completely and understandably? Are the office staff friendly and helpful? Is this a person I can talk to about intimate details of my life? Is there likely to be a clash of egos?

How do I go about finding a doctor after a move or when traveling? Before moving, ask your doctor to recommend a doctor in your new locale. If your doctor does not have a recommendation, consult the local medical society, medical center, or teaching hospital for a list of names. After you have some names, go through the screening process outlined earlier.

If an urgent problem develops while traveling, go to the nearest emergency room. Cruise ships and many large hotels have staff doctors or can call one for you. If you are planning an extended stay abroad, most American consulate offices can provide lists of local physicians. (See Chapter 14 for precautions to take while traveling.)

I'm unhappy with my present arrangement. How do I go about changing doctors? Even the most careful selection process sometimes ends up with a poor fit. If after a few visits you feel this isn't the right doctor or office for you, don't feel you must stay. Many people put their doctors on a pedestal, hesitating to question or voice their unhappiness with the manner in which they are being treated. They are likely to feel guilty about changing doctors, even if they know the relationship is not working. But remember, the doctor's job is to work with you to help you be well. Just as you can switch a lawyer or accountant, so too can you change doctors.

Before deciding to change, however, ask yourself if you are harboring unrealistic expectations. Indeed, you may be part of the problem, especially if you find yourself going from doctor to doctor in search of one who will tell you only what you want to hear. Sometimes too a doctor-patient problem is one of poor communication, so before making a switch, try a frank discussion of your concerns. As in any interpersonal relationship, talking through a problem can sometimes produce a solution. If this doesn't help, however, you may be better off finding a more compatible fit. Start the process anew, and after you've found a new doctor, ask your former one to forward your medical records. Your former doctor's office staff will generally ask you to sign a release form before they transfer their records to another health-care provider.

SUMMING UP

Any effective heart-care program requires a careful evaluation of your individual situation. The goal is to increase your odds for a healthy future by defining your risks and considering the benefits of lifestyle changes and, if needed, treatment. Your mindset is critical; so too is the attitude of your spouse or companion. Your long-term success is a matter of finding the strategies for heart health that will work best for you. The following chapters address how to create a balanced, individualized approach that can be sustained for a lifetime.

I

Lifestyle
and
Heart
Health

A prudent lifestyle is critical for achieving and maintaining good health, especially when it comes to benefiting the heart. How many times has your doctor advised you to exercise more, eat less, reduce stress, and—if you smoke—stop? If you're a typical American, the answer is probably almost every time you see your doctor. You leave the office determined to change, and you make a serious effort to do so, only to find that after a few weeks you have slipped back into the same old sedentary, fast-food, stressed-out rut.

Why is it so hard to adopt a more healthful lifestyle, especially when you know it may help avoid heart disease and extend your life? There's no easy answer, but we can identify some of the more common pitfalls.

MAKING TOO MANY CHANGES AT ONCE

Attempting a sea change in lifestyle is especially prevalent among persons who have suffered a heart attack or some other life-threatening event. Fear, especially after a close call with death, is a great initial motivator. Heart patients invariably leave the hospital determined to "shape up," and for a time, most make many changes to become more healthy. But eventually the fear factor wanes, and within a year or so, many patients will have reverted to their former ways. Sadly, more than a few of these patients will suffer another life-threatening—or life-ending—episode.

How can patients sustain not just their good intentions, but also their positive lifestyle changes? First, remember you are developing a program that will benefit you for the rest of your life. Just as the condition didn't develop overnight, so too you cannot develop immediately the optimal lifestyle to combat it. Take the case of Stanley. This fifty-five-year-old executive readily admits that he's hard-driving, often working twelve or more hours a day, six or seven days a week. He travels a good deal, taking many of his meals in restaurants without paying much attention to his doctor's dietary guidelines. His LDL (bad) cholesterol is too high, as is his blood pressure. His doctor had prescribed medication for both, but he often takes the drugs only now and then, frequently forgetting to pack them when he travels, which is often two or three days a week.

After a heart attack and successful coronary artery bypass surgery, Stanley left the hospital vowing to change all this and more. He enrolled in a cardiac rehab program, which emphasized exercise, diet, and stress management. With great determination, he joined a gym and signed on with a personal trainer. The eating plan recommended by the rehab dietitian wasn't producing the fast results he craved, so he put himself on the latest low-fat, low-carb diet. He dropped twenty-two of his excess fifty pounds in the first month. He tried cutting his work schedule by assigning some of his travel to a junior associate.

All went well for a few months, but then the daily treadmill workouts exacerbated the arthritis in his knees, so he decided to skip a few sessions at the gym. Somehow he never got back into the exercise routine. Then a downturn in his business prompted him to step up his work schedule and resume traveling at least three days a week to visit clients. He found it impossible to stick to his strict low-carb diet when entertaining clients and his favorite restaurants didn't offer the low-fat selections mandated by his diet. So this, too, went by the boards. He still forgot to pack his medication, so he again was taking his pills intermittently.

By the time Stanley went for his six-month post-bypass checkup, his weight was back to its former level and his blood pressure and cholesterol were again elevated, probably because he wasn't taking his medication every day. His doctor warned Stanley that he was headed for another heart attack and offered to help him work out a more realistic lifelong regimen. After a few hits and misses, the two came up with a program that took into account Stanley's driven mindset, work, arthritic knees, dietary preferences, and propensity to forget his blood pressure and cholesterol-lowering medications. (Details about his regimen and his success in living it are described in Chapter 2.)

COEXISTING DISORDERS

Stanley cited his chronic knee problems as a reason for stopping his daily exercise program. Arthritis and other orthopedic problems are common hindrances, but they are not the only disorders that can complicate developing an exercise program and adopting other lifestyle changes. Alice, the forty-five-year-old part-time school aide, is markedly obese and also has type II diabetes. After suffering a major heart attack, she realized it was imperative that she increase her exercise and lose weight. But her efforts were complicated by her diabetes, which had caused leg and foot problems. She was also fearful that exercise would bring on another heart attack.

Asthma and other pulmonary problems are other common disorders that hamper efforts to exercise. Even so, these coexisting disorders are obstacles that can be overcome. With proper planning and adjustments, virtually everyone can utilize some form of a heart-healthy exercise program. Exercising in water, for example, takes the pressure off arthritic joints; and people with pulmonary disorders almost always can undertake a graduated program that accommodates, and may even improve, their lung function.

PSYCHOLOGICAL ROADBLOCKS

After a heart attack, many people are afraid to exercise because they mistakenly believe it can cause another heart attack. In fact, the opposite is true: a well-designed exercise program can both improve cardiovascular fitness and at least partially protect against another heart attack. People suffering from depression often find it difficult to summon up the energy to exercise or make other lifestyle changes. Anxiety and panic attacks can also make exercise difficult. Yet these too are challenges that, once identified and then overcome, are actually themselves improved by regular exercise.

DENIAL OF DEVELOPING OR POTENTIAL PROBLEMS

"Don't tell me, I don't want to know!" or "I'm so healthy, how can anything be wrong?" These are all-too-common roadblocks to instituting lifestyle changes. Jennifer, the fifty-year-old runner introduced earlier, is a prime example. She was trim, muscular, and the very picture of fitness and good health. But her strong family history of early heart attacks increased her risk of developing some form of cardiovascular disease. When she started experiencing unusual chest pains after running, she at first denied she could be developing heart disease. So it took several months and a steady worsening of her symptoms before she saw a doctor. Even so, she was stunned to learn that she had advanced coronary artery disease and was at high risk of suffering a heart attack. Luckily, an interventional cardiology procedure—angioplasty to open her clogged coronary arteries and insertion of a device (stent) to keep them open—was successful. Before long, she was again running, although at a more moderate level than before. (Her treatment and outcome are discussed more fully in Chapter 2.)

GEOGRAPHIC, CULTURAL, AND ECONOMIC FACTORS

Doctors hear dozens of excuses for not exercising or adopting other lifestyle changes. "I just don't have the time." "I can't afford to join a gym or to buy expensive exercise machines." "I don't have a safe place where I can walk." "I have to eat what I feed my children and all they want are hotdogs, burgers, and French fries." "I'm afraid I'll get fat if I stop smoking." Perhaps you can echo one or more of these, and no doubt we can all add others.

In the final analysis, however, these are only excuses, and all can be overcome with the right attitude and a commonsense approach. Learning about yourself—what puts you in the mainstream of patients, as well as what makes you different—will help set you on the path toward both of these goals. The chapters in Part I provide specific guidelines for getting started on a workable lifestyle program, and, more importantly, how to adopt it for life.

CHAPTER

2

Exercise Your Way to a Healthy
Heart and Body

Hundreds of scientific studies document the long-term benefits of regular exercise. These include increased longevity in both men and women and a markedly reduced risk of developing cardiovascular disease and type II diabetes. Regular exercise can produce modest reductions in blood pressure and total cholesterol, LDL (the bad cholesterol), and triglycerides (another blood lipid), while raising levels of HDL (the good cholesterol). (People who have significantly elevated cholesterol and high blood pressure, however, usually need medication in addition to exercise and dietary changes to bring these problems under control.)

Heart attack patients especially benefit from regular exercise. A statistical review of twenty-two different studies that followed more than four thousand patients for three years found that the death rate among patients who had participated in a cardiac rehab program that included regular exercise was 20 to 25 percent lower than among those whose program did not include the exercise training. Other studies conducted over the last twenty years have found an improvement in cardiovascular symptoms among heart patients who engaged in regular exercise. These improvements included increased endurance in persons with heart failure, a lessening of chest pains (angina), and a reduction in leg pain caused by reduced blood flow to the leg muscles (intermittent claudication).

Still other studies have documented improved heart function among both patients with cardiovascular disease and healthy individuals who engage in aerobic exercise (such as walking, jogging, or cycling). Maximum benefits are achieved by persons who exercise for thirty minutes at least three to five days a week and at an intensity suitable for their condition (see Box 3). These benefits include a more efficient uptake of oxygen during exercise, an increase in the amount of blood pumped out with each heartbeat (stroke volume), and a lower resting heart rate, which reduces the heart's overall workload. Exercise conditioning enables the muscles to use oxygen more efficiently, further reducing the workload of the heart. Regular exercise also helps mitigate age-related changes in cardiovascular function and increases stamina.

Of course, the benefits of regular exercise are by no means limited to cardiovascular health. Exercise is an important component in managing diabetes because it helps the body make more efficient use of insulin, the hormone essential for proper metabolism of carbohydrates. Weight-bearing exercise is a critical component of building and maintaining healthy bones and, as such, can help prevent or slow the progression of osteoporosis. Exercise can be a major modifier of stress; it also promotes an enhanced sense of well-being and improved self-image. It is an effective treatment for some types of depression, especially when combined with other treatments. Exercise increases levels of endorphins, the body's natural painkillers. And regular exercise fights obesity in two ways—it helps burn excess calories and helps prevent overeating by controlling appetite.

TEN SIMPLE RULES FOR A SUCCESSFUL EXERCISE PROGRAM

1. *Your exercise regimen should change as your life circumstances change.* We can't overemphasize the importance of developing a lifelong commitment to regular exercise. But activities that are well suited for a thirty-year-old may not be appropriate for persons in their seventies or eighties. Similarly, changes in health may mandate adjustments in an exercise regimen. This is what happened to Jennifer, the fifty-year-old long-distance runner introduced earlier. Running had been an important part of her life since she was a teenager, but after several months of worsening chest pains after a run, she saw her doctor. Both of Jennifer's parents had suffered heart attacks in their early sixties, and her fifty-four-year-old brother had recently undergone coronary bypass surgery. An exercise stress test with imaging, followed by angiography, confirmed that Jennifer had moderately severe

Box 3

DETERMINING YOUR SAFE AND EFFECTIVE HEART RATE DURING EXERCISE

To determine your heart rate:

- Press two fingers of one hand on the artery on the inside of your wrist or the carotid artery, located under the jaw on either side of the front of the neck.
- Using a stopwatch, count the pulse beats for fifteen seconds.
- Multiply the result by four to determine your total beats per minute.
- During exercise, stop briefly to take your pulse after you have exercised for a few minutes at your peak intensity. (You can also buy a heart-rate monitor, available in most stores that sell exercise equipment, to wear while exercising. These simple devices often involve strapping a small monitor around your chest. The heart rate is typically displayed digitally on a bracelet or wristwatch-like device. Similarly, treadmills and many other exercise machines automatically monitor pulse rate.)

To determine your maximum heart rate (beats per minute), subtract your age from 220.

- Example: If you are 55 years old, 220 minus 55 = 165 (maximum heart rate)

To determine your target heart rate during exercise:

- If you have been sedentary, start by aiming for 50 to 60 percent of your maximum heart rate. (For example, if your maximum rate is 165 beats per minute, aim for a range of 82 to 99 beats per minute.)
- If you are a healthy adult, aim for a heart rate of 60 to 85 percent of your maximum heart rate. (For example, if your maximum heart rate is 165 beats per minute, aim for a range of 99 to 140 beats per minute.) You may increase your heart-rate goal as you continue exercising and increase your stamina.
- If you have established cardiovascular risk factors (for example, you smoke, are overweight, or have high blood pressure, elevated cholesterol, or diabetes) aim for a heart rate of 55 to 75 percent of your maximum. (For example, if your maximum heart rate is 165, aim for a range of 90 to 123.) Remember, maximum heart rates are based on average values. There are many individual exceptions that will require adjustments to these age-defined levels.

(*continued*)

(Box 3 *continued*)

- Persons with known heart disease and ischemia or chest pain (angina) should have an exercise stress test before undertaking any exercise regimen, and that program should follow a doctor's individualized exercise prescription. The doctor will require that the patient stop exercising below the heart rate that provokes ischemia or chest pain. For example, if symptoms develop at a heart rate of 130 beats per minute, the person may be instructed to exercise only to a rate of 110 beats per minute.

Important: Your doctor may advise you to aim for a lower target heart rate depending on your individual risk factors and other circumstances. You may also be advised to have an exercise stress test before beginning an exercise program to determine your safe heart rate. Always follow your doctor's instructions, and stop exercising immediately if you experience dizziness, chest pain, shortness of breath, or other serious symptoms. If the symptoms do not abate in a few minutes, seek immediate medical attention by calling 911 or your local emergency medical services.

coronary artery disease. Although she probably could have controlled it with medication, diet, and less intensive exercise, in view of her active lifestyle and life goals, her doctor advised that she undergo angioplasty. In this common medical procedure, a balloon-tipped catheter is inserted into the clogged coronary artery. After the balloon is inflated to flatten the plaque, a tiny umbrella-shaped device called a stent is inserted to help keep the artery open. (See Chapter 7 for details about this procedure.)

After her treatment, Jennifer gradually resumed her exercise regimen, starting at a more moderate pace than in the past by alternating brisk walking and cycling with shorter runs. She also decided to forgo running in marathons in favor of an occasional 5K or 10K event. By tailoring her exercise regimen to reduce her risk for heart injury, she was able to continue to enjoy her active lifestyle without further endangering her heart or suffering chest pain.

2. *Accept no excuses for not getting started.* Virtually everyone can undertake an exercise program, regardless of age, health, work schedule, and other circumstances. Studies show that even people in their eighties and nineties, including those confined to wheelchairs or nursing homes, can benefit from an exercise program—although the exercises they do may

look different from those most younger people try. The same is true of people with severe heart disease and other medical problems. After her severe heart attack, Alice, the forty-five-year-old mother of three, felt that exercise was dangerous, if not impossible, until she enrolled in a cardiac rehab program. An exercise physiologist designed a regimen for Alice that started with walking ten to fifteen minutes a day, which she worked into her busy schedule by making it a family endeavor. Instead of parking near the school where she worked part-time and where two of her children were students, she parked a few blocks away and the three then walked the rest of the way. The return walk in the afternoon gave her a second fifteen-minute walk and an opportunity to spend more time chatting with her children. As her fitness improved, she lengthened the walking time and, two or three times a week, used one of her breaks to lift weights with a group of teachers in the school gym.

Alice is a prime example of a very busy person who can find time to exercise and—more important—can enjoy the experience. No matter how busy you are, you can find time to exercise the recommended four or five times a week. For example, you can position a stationary bike, treadmill, or other machine in front of the TV and exercise while you watch the news or one of your favorite programs. Or you can get up a half-hour earlier and enjoy an outdoor jog or walk before breakfast. Stop making excuses and start moving!

3. *Build your regimen around activities you enjoy.* No matter how motivated you are, chances are you'll give up if exercise is more chore than pleasure. If you hate jogging, there's little point in making it the center-piece of your regimen. In contrast, if you truly enjoy walking your dog, get your exercise by setting a brisker pace and going a bit farther than usual. Chances are both you and your dog will benefit. If you prefer exercising with others, link up with a mall-walking group or join an exercise class at your local gym, "Y," school, or senior center. Swimming and water aerobics are excellent forms of exercise, although they require access to a pool or beach. Variety is key. To avoid boredom, try varying your routine; perhaps walking or jogging two or three times a week, swing dancing or an aerobics class once a week, and swimming, working out at a gym, or enrolling in an exercise class on the other day(s).

4. *Invest in the proper equipment.* You don't need to spend thousands to equip a home gym to achieve physical and cardiovascular fitness, but at the very least, you need the proper shoes, especially if your regimen is built

around running, jogging, or walking (see Box 4). Your exercise garb should be comfortable and appropriate for the weather. If you exercise outdoors when it's cold, wear lightweight insulated exercise clothes, and if you are walking or jogging at night or early morning, be sure to wear reflective material to make yourself more visible to motorists.

If you do buy exercise equipment, look for models that are sturdy and easy to use and be sure to try them out before buying. In fact, it's a good idea to go to a gym and engage a trainer for a session or two to let you try out a variety of machines and show you how to use them properly. Pick equipment that you truly enjoy; otherwise that fancy treadmill or exercise cycle is likely to become a clotheshorse rather than a fun way to work out.

Your exercise regimen should also include strength training, which is essential to achieve good muscle tone and maintain healthy bones; it also helps improve balance, maintain proper metabolism and weight, and foster a sense of well-being. Strength training can be done at a gym or weight room or at home with a simple set of free weights (for most people, five-, ten-, and fifteen-pound weights are sufficient). A length of surgical tubing or set of Therabands, both used to provide resistance, help tone muscles and increase strength. If you travel frequently, seek out hotels that have health clubs (most now do). Many commercial gyms or health clubs also have reciprocal arrangements with facilities in other cities; you might check to see if your home membership will allow you to exercise for free in another location.

Stretching is also an important element in an exercise regimen, and a good floor mat makes this component more comfortable and easier to carry out. Do not attempt to stretch at the beginning of a workout, however; instead, stretch at the end, when muscles are warmed up and less susceptible to injury. Start slowly and stretch with smooth, easy movements.

5. *If you are sedentary, start slowly and build gradually.* It has probably taken you years of sedentary living to reach your present state, so it's unrealistic to expect to become fit after only a few weeks or even months of exercise. All too many sedentary individuals make the mistake of doing too much too fast and then end up sidelined by aches or injury. We typically recommend starting slowly, perhaps with ten or fifteen minutes of walking at a moderate pace five or more times a week. Then over a period of weeks or months, increase the intensity and duration of the exercise until you achieve your target heart rate and level of fitness. You can then embark on a maintenance program and vary your exercises to increase your enjoyment

Box 4

MAKE SURE THE SHOE FITS

Many exercise-related muscle and orthopedic problems actually origi-nate in the feet. This is why it's essential that your shoes match your chosen activity. Here are a few pointers:

- *Replace athletic shoes as needed.* Walking or jogging shoes should be re-placed every five hundred miles or so. If in doubt, set the shoes on a flat surface and look at them from the back. If they lean inward or outward or show signs of wear on the soles' edges, it's time to get new shoes.

- *Make sure the shoes fit properly.* When buying your first pair, it's a good idea to go to a sports store that has salespeople experienced in fitting ath-letic shoes. Buy new shoes after a workout or at the end of the day when your feet are their largest. Be sure to wear the same socks that you wear during a workout. Make sure you can wiggle all your toes freely. When try-ing on a new pair, walk or run a few steps in them. Some stores even have treadmills for this purpose. Shoes should be comfortable from the start; they shouldn't need "breaking in" to feel good on your feet: in particular, your heel should not slip and the sole should both provide good traction and be flexible enough to allow the foot to roll properly with each step.

- *Make sure that the shoes accommodate any foot problems.* If you have flat feet or tend to roll your feet inward (pronate) when you walk or run, look for shoes with added arch support. Try several different brands and select the ones that best meet your needs. For example, if you walk with toes pointed out or have high arches, look for shoes with extra cushioning. If you use orthotics or special insoles, make sure the toe box is deep enough to accommodate them. Pay special attention to heel stability, and reject any that allow the heel to slip up and down in the shoe.

If you participate in an activity three or more times a week, you probably need shoes designed specifically for that sport. Here are common examples of activity-specific shoes:

- *Walking.* Shoes should be lightweight with good arch supports and wide enough to accommodate the ball of the foot. Heels should be padded, wide, and close to the ground to provide stability; some walking shoes have built-in contoured heel stabilizers. A molded inner heel and beveled outer "rocker sole" promote proper foot roll-through with each step. Make sure the upper back does not touch the ankle bones or "bite" into the heel. Soles should be of a shock-absorbent material, such as polyurethane, and

(continued)

(Box 4 *continued*)

scored to provide good traction. The uppers should be of leather, mesh, or another "breathable" material and flexible enough to allow the foot to move properly.

- *Running.* Shoes should be fully flexible at the ball of the foot, with padded soles to absorb the impact of running. The soles should provide enough traction to prevent slipping. Good arch supports are essential, and runners with problem feet may need orthotic devices to provide extra support and prevent pronation, the inward rolling of the foot. Again, try different brands until you find one that works for you.

- *Cross-training.* Good walking shoes can double for cross-training. Special cross-trainers combine features of both walking and running shoes; look for models that are comfortable and suited to your specific regimen.

- *Cycling.* Look for shoes that provide rigid support across the arch; a heel lift may also be needed. Long-distance cyclists may need toe clips or special cleats to prevent the foot from slipping off the pedals.

- *Hiking.* Shoes should be sturdy with high tops to provide firm ankle support. Soles may be studded or scored to provide extra traction. Make sure the toe boxes are roomy enough to accommodate thick, absorbent socks.

- *Tennis.* Shoes should be lightweight and made of canvas or other breathable material. The toe box should be padded; the shoe should also have arch supports and be flexible enough to allow side-to-side sliding. Heels should be cushioned and fit snugly; look for low-traction soles.

- *Field sports, such as soccer, football, or track and field.* Depending on the sport, the shoes may have cleats, studs, or other devices. The key is to look for shoes that provide proper ankle support.

Important: Don't scrimp on the cost; good shoes are a sound investment in your fitness program. Go to a shoe store that specializes in fitting athletic shoes. Once you know your proper size, style, and favorite brand, you may be able to save money by ordering from a catalogue or on-line store.

Remember, too, that your socks deserve almost as much attention as your shoes, especially if you have diabetes or circulatory problems. The socks should be made of an absorbent material that wicks moisture away from the skin. They should fit the foot snugly without bunching, wrinkling, or binding. Discard any socks that have holes. Avoid those that have tight elastic tops because they can cut blood flow; if you have varicose veins or impaired leg circulation, consider wearing special support socks.

and continue improving your health. (Near the end of this chapter, we discuss a model program that can be adapted to meet your personal needs.)

Some people thrive on competitive sports, but avoid becoming a "weekend warrior"; exercising once or twice a week is not enough. In fact, if that's all you do, you have a higher risk of injuries, such as twisting a knee, suffering a tennis elbow, or rupturing an Achilles tendon. So instead of (or in addition to) a vigorous game of handball or tennis once a week, it's better to fill in the other days with a workout on a treadmill, exercise cycle, elliptical trainer, or other activity. Remember, too, that your goal is physical and cardiovascular fitness, not becoming a world-class athlete.

6. *Respect injuries and illness.* Some muscle stiffness and minor aches may occur when you first embark on an exercise program or increase its intensity or duration, but they should not be chronic conditions. Forget what you've heard about "No pain, no gain." Exercise, weight training, and stretching should not cause pain. Indeed, most exercise-related injuries are due to overuse of fatigued muscles and joints or undertaking too much exercise too quickly. If you experience exercise-related pain or injury, don't ignore it. Joint, tendon, and muscle injuries are especially common among joggers and runners, and should be treated as soon as possible. In fact, continuing to exercise when you are injured can exacerbate the problem and sideline you even longer. Simple overuse injuries usually heal with rest. (You can switch to other low-impact activities during this time.) If the problem persists, see a doctor or exercise physiologist to determine the precise cause. Very often, ankle, knee, hip, and back problems actually originate in the feet, and are best treated by a podiatrist or orthopedist who specializes in dealing with athletic injuries. Sometimes simple foot problems can be corrected by switching shoes or using orthotics, devices that are fitted into shoes to give extra arch support or cushioning help correct a faulty gait. Nonprescription orthotic devices may be sufficient; but more often, the best results come from investing in prescription devices designed by an exercise podiatrist or trainer for your particular feet.

It may take several weeks to get over a viral illness, such as flu or bronchitis. Respect these transient illnesses and reduce your exercising or stop completely until you feel totally recovered.

Illnesses and injuries occur even in an appropriate exercise regimen. But stopping your exercise to attend to an injury should be only a temporary setback. Restart your exercise when you are ready, and when you do, remember that this is a plan for life; as you recover, slowly reinstitute your activity and gradually work back up to your former level and goals. This may take several weeks. Be patient: it will take time to regain your former stamina.

7. *Build cross training and variety into your regimen.* Cross training—varying your regimen by rotating among different aerobic, flexibility, and strengthening exercises—helps avoid injuries. When you vary your aerobic activities (for example, if you jog on day one, then cycle or swim on day two), you are giving the parts of your body stressed by the jogging a chance to recover while placing stress on different parts of your anatomy the next day. Variety also fights the boredom of doing the same routine over and over, week in and week out. We've touched on this point before, but it bears repeating: Variety is just as important in an exercise program as in other facets of life. And in our personal regimens, we've found that cross training has become even more important as we age.

Your choice of activities also should be related to your health. For example, if you have bad knees, jogging and running are not good choices; instead, look for low-impact activities such as walking, swimming, low-impact aerobic dancing, cross-country skiing or ski machines, or elliptical trainers. Varying your activities also helps minimize your risk of exercise-related injuries.

8. *Remember to warm up before—and stretch after—exercise, and be sure to include flexibility and strength training.* Do not stretch or exercise cold muscles; this practice greatly increases the chance of injury. Instead, warm up with a few minutes of walking or other mild activity to increase blood flow to the muscles and "warm them up." Five minutes is usually enough. You are then ready to increase your activity level to achieve your target heart rate and endurance goal. After exercising in your peak range, cool down gradually by repeating the warm-up activity. You are then ready to conclude the session with a few minutes of stretching or flexibility exercises. You should include stretching exercises for all of your major muscles and joints, including specific stretches for your problem areas. For example, if you are bothered by back pain, be sure to include stretching exercises that are designed for the back.

9. *Drink water during and after exercise.* It is important to drink enough water to replace the body fluids lost in perspiration. Maintaining proper hydration is especially important during prolonged exercise and during hot, humid weather. It's a good idea to carry a bottle of water with you and to take frequent sips throughout the session. Practice moderation, how-

ever; a 2005 report in the *New England Journal of Medicine* described a number of serious problems, including brain swelling and even death, among marathon runners who consumed too much water during a race. The excessive water upsets the body's balance of sodium and other electrolytes. Your goal should be simply to replace the fluids you lose while perspiring without overloading the body with water.

Some people recommend sports drinks that include salts to replace the electrolytes lost when sweating. In most circumstances, however, plain water is just as adequate. Many sports drinks, as well as sodas and fruit juices, are high in calories. So if you enjoy a couple of glasses of orange juice after a workout, you may be adding back many of the calories you've just burned off. In addition, sipping water or sports drinks flavored with acidic substances can harm tooth enamel. If you favor these flavored liquids, drink them quickly to avoid prolonged contact with the teeth.

10. *Use common sense.* Safety is just as important as the exercise itself. If you jog or walk along a road, always stay well to the side, facing the traffic for a better view, and pay attention to your surroundings. Headphones may be distracting because they block out traffic noise and other warnings. Wear reflective clothing at night and avoid dark streets and deserted parks or other places where you might be confronted or harmed. And don't approach strange dogs. When traveling, if you're unsure about the safety of a park or area, ask a local resident for advice. Hotels can provide maps or advise you of a safe route; if in doubt, work out in the hotel's health club or at a nearby gym. If you have heart disease, diabetes, severe allergies, or another potentially serious medical condition, wear a MedicAlert bracelet that can provide details about your condition to emergency personnel. Also, carry some sort of identification, perhaps a cell phone, and enough money to hail a cab in an emergency.

THE FUNDAMENTALS OF EXERCISE AND FITNESS

In general, physical fitness is measured in terms of endurance as well as the body's ability to use oxygen efficiently and to convert enough carbohydrates and other nutrients into energy. Other components include muscular strength and flexibility, as well as the ratio of lean body tissue to fat. Numerous studies have shown that burning two thousand calories a week through exercise not only maintains fitness but also extends life. (Table 1 lists the calories expended during common activities.)

TABLE 1

CALORIES USED IN VARIOUS ACTIVITIES

Activity	Calories burned per minute
Bicycling, 6 mph	4
Bicycling, 10 mph	7
Bicycling, 12 mph	9
Canoeing, 2.5 mph	4
Dancing, aerobic	9
Dancing, ballroom or square	6
Gardening	4
Golfing, pulling cart	5
Ice skating	7
Jogging, 5 mph	8
Jogging, 7 mph	12
Jumping rope, slow	7
Jumping rope, medium	9
Jumping rope, fast	11
Roller-skating	6
Rowing, machine	6
Rowing, scull racing	7
Running, 8 mph	13
Running, 10 mph	17
Skiing, cross-country	11
Skiing, downhill, 10 mph	10
Squash or handball	10
Table tennis	6
Tennis, singles	7
Tennis, doubles	6
Walking, 2 mph	3
Walking, 3 mph	5
Walking, 4 mph	7

Note: *the number of calories is calculated for a 150-pound person. Because individual metabolic rates vary, all numbers are approximate, but they are useful in establishing relative values of various activities.*

Source: Adapted from B. L. Zaret, M. Moser, and L. S. Cohen, eds., *Yale University School of Medicine Heart Book* (New York: Hearst Books, 1992).

Types of Exercise

There are two basic types of exercise: *aerobic,* which increases the muscles' need for oxygen, and *anaerobic* (also referred to as *resistance* or *isometric* exercise), which does not require the muscles to burn extra oxygen. Examples of aerobic exercise include low- to moderate-impact activities such as brisk walking, step aerobics, rowing, swimming, cross-country skiing, and swimming. High-impact aerobic activities include jogging, running, racquetball, squash, and singles tennis. Such high-impact activities tend to burn calories more quickly than low-impact exercises do, but they also carry a greater risk of muscle, joint, and tendon injuries. Regardless of the type, regular aerobic exercise increases endurance and improves cardiovascular function, provided it is done regularly (at least four or fives times a week) and at sufficient intensity and duration.

Anaerobic activities include weight-lifting, some types of calisthenics, and the use of resistance exercise machines. These activities build muscle mass and strength, improve balance, and help maintain bones—all important benefits for older persons.

The Three Variables of Every Exercise Program

Three variables influence the beneficial or training effect of exercise: frequency, duration, and intensity. Aerobic activities that require moderate exertion over an extended period are the most effective for improving cardiovascular function.

To obtain maximum benefits, we recommend that you exercise for an average of thirty minutes three to five days a week. (You may exercise longer or more frequently provided that doing so does not provoke symptoms or complications.) The more intensive the exercise, the greater the cardiovascular conditioning. Most healthy adults should strive for five weekly sessions, and those who need to lose weight should plan five or six low-impact workouts a week. (As a general rule, you should refrain from exercise one or two days a week to give the body a chance to recover.) The duration varies according to individual factors and the type of exercise. A sedentary person just starting a regimen may be well advised to start with one or two ten-minute sessions three times a week and to gradually increase the intensity and duration as endurance improves. The type of exercise also influences how long you should exercise. Walking or jogging a mile burns about a hundred calories, regardless of how fast or slow you go. For example, walking a mile in twenty minutes burns the same number of calories as running a mile in ten minutes. Thus, if the goal is to burn three hundred calories, you can achieve this in a half hour of running at a rate of six miles per hour, or an hour of walking at three miles per hour.

As for intensity, the goal is to exercise at a certain percentage of your maximum safe heart rate, depending on your general health, age, and cardiovascular risk factors (see Box 3). In general, an obese or older person should exercise at a more moderate pace; for example, start at 50 or 55 percent of the maximum safe heart rate and gradually increase this over time. You'll soon learn what is comfortable for you. As a rule of thumb, many experts recommend adopting a "talking pace," which is intense enough to raise your heart rate and produce sweating but moderate enough that you can carry on a conversation without gasping for breath. At first, you may be able to achieve this pace only while walking at a moderate pace, but as your fitness and endurance improve, you'll be able to pick up the pace without feeling out of breath.

Warming up before exercise and cooling down afterward will help avoid injury and discomfort. We recommend five to ten minutes of warm-up exercises—for example, walking at a moderate pace, swinging the arms, or slow jogging in place—at the beginning of each session. An older person may need an even longer warm-up. Some people do stretches during their warm-up, but do so with great caution, if at all, because stretching cold muscles increases the risk of injury. How you conclude an exercise session is also important because stopping abruptly can result in muscle cramps and/or a drop in blood pressure and dizziness, especially in older persons. So at the end of the session take five or ten minutes (or longer if you wish) to cool down by exercising gently—for example, walking at a slow pace—until your heart rate is again ten to fifteen beats a minute faster than your normal resting pulse. Gentle stretching exercises should also be part of the cooldown period.

DESIGNING YOUR PERSONALIZED EXERCISE PROGRAM

Just as no one treatment program fits all, so too there's no single exercise regimen that's appropriate for everyone. But there are some common denominators. We've already discussed some of these—namely, lifelong commitment, frequency, intensity, duration, and variety. When it comes to designing your own program, there are at least three important questions to be answered.

1. *Do I need my doctor's okay before starting?* In general, a pre-exercise medical checkup is not necessary for healthy persons under the age of forty if they are free of cardiovascular risk factors. Of course, this leaves a

vast number of people who should see a doctor first. Specifically, the American Heart Association recommends a checkup that includes an exercise stress test, and perhaps other studies depending on individual circumstances, for anyone over the age of forty who has had a heart attack or has symptoms or a family history of coronary artery disease. The same recommendation is made for anyone over age forty who has two or more of the cardiovascular risk factors outlined in Chapter 1. A checkup may also be in order for younger people who have one or two risk factors or who plan to undertake a new, strenuous activity such as cross-country skiing or long-distance running. Testing may also be recommended for people who are very sedentary, as well as those over the age of sixty or sixty-five, even though they are free of symptoms or known risk factors. If in doubt, check with your doctor before starting an exercise program. (See Box 5 for further cautions regarding exercise programs.)

2. *How do I establish goals that are best for me?* Obviously, goals vary greatly from one person to another. Some people simply want to get in shape, increase endurance and strength, or lose a few pounds—all important goals for establishing and maintaining good health. Others may undertake an exercise program to achieve specific health benefits or to reduce or eliminate cardiovascular risk factors. For example, regular exercise is a critical component of managing diabetes; it can also help lower blood pressure and produce modest increases in HDL (good) cholesterol.

Regardless of specific health-related goals, any exercise program should include both aerobic (endurance-building) and anaerobic (resistance or strengthening) activities. As noted earlier, most sedentary people need to start at a low level and build up gradually as strength and endurance increase. Ideally, the aerobic activity should be done for thirty to sixty minutes four to six times a week and be intense enough to burn at least two thousand calories a week (see Table 1). The resistance exercises should be done two or three times a week and include ten to fifteen repetitions a set, for eight to ten sets, of exercises designed to strengthen specific muscle groups (arms, shoulders, chest, trunk, back, hips, and legs). Strengthening exercises should be designed to improve tone rather than build muscle. Many women shun weight training because they fear developing bulging muscles. In reality, as muscles become stronger and toned, the body looks trimmer, not "bulked up." Also, well-toned muscle tissue is more metabolically active and will help with weight control even when you are not exercising.

Exercise activity can also be expressed as metabolic equivalents (METs), a term commonly used by medical professionals prescribing an exercise program. METs are used to measure the amount of oxygen consumed by a person at rest (one MET is the metabolic rate that occurs when 3.5 milliliters of oxygen a minute are consumed per kilogram of body weight). Multiples of this value are a useful way to indicate the level of energy used during exercise. For example, doing gardening generally uses three to five METs, whereas jogging uses seven to fifteen METs.

3. *When is it safe to start exercising after a heart attack?* Depending on the severity of the heart attack, type of treatment, and other individual factors, most doctors recommend resuming moderate physical activity—sitting in a chair, standing, walking—as soon as the patient is stabilized. Following discharge from the hospital, at a time determined by your doctor and based on the type of heart attack, complications, and treatment, cardiac rehabilitation that includes an exercise program is strongly recommended for almost all patients. A stress test is usually required before beginning exercise. (See Chapter 6.) Typically, the patient starts exercising under the supervision of an exercise physiologist, nurse, or other professional. Group exercise is especially beneficial because patients can encourage one another and understand that they are not alone.

After safe parameters are established, the patient can start working out without supervision. Still, some caution is advised. Obviously, you should stop and rest if you experience symptoms of possible cardiovascular origin, such as chest pain (angina), light-headedness, nausea or vomiting, pallor, shortness of breath, and palpitations or a racing heartbeat. (Seek immediate medical help if these symptoms persist after more than a few minutes of rest.)

A MODEL EXERCISE PROGRAM: WHAT WORKED FOR STANLEY

There is no model program that works for everyone; instead, find activities that you can enjoy doing long-term and then design a program to meet your individual goals. Still, it can be useful to learn what exercise regimens have been prescribed for others, such as Stanley, the fifty-five-year-old executive who suffered a mild heart attack and then underwent coronary bypass surgery. His program was developed during his enrollment in a cardiac rehab program, during his recovery phase. In his first week, he was told to walk for five to ten minutes with his heart rate at 50 percent of his maximum safe rate (80 to 85 beats a minute)

Box 5

STAYING ON TRACK: EXERCISE TROUBLESHOOTING

Although it's important to make exercise an integral part of your daily routine, there are times when you should lay off or use special caution. In this regard, let common sense be your guide.

Weather. Pay attention to weather reports, and act accordingly. If the weather is very hot and humid, work out or walk in an indoor, air-conditioned environment, such as a gym or enclosed mall. Similarly, avoid exercising outdoors when it's very cold or icy underfoot, especially if the cold provokes chest pains, breathing problems (such as asthma), or other symptoms. In either instance, dress appropriately.

Changes in altitude. Also use caution if you're going from a low altitude to one that's higher than four thousand feet (see Chapter 14). Give your body a few days to get used to the "thinner" air before working out. Even then, be alert to any warning symptoms such as light-headedness, dizziness, shortness of breath, fatigue, or headaches.

Travel. A business or pleasure trip is no excuse to stop exercising. Most hotels have an exercise room or pool that guests can use, and most commercial gyms will welcome visitors for a modest fee. If you are a jogger or walker, pack the appropriate shoes and workout garb and ask the concierge or desk clerk to suggest a safe and convenient place where you can walk or jog. For resistance training, work out in the hotel health club or, if you prefer, pack a length of surgical tubing or Therabands to use in lieu of free weights.

After an illness. If you've been laid up with a bad cold or bout of flu, chances are you've had to temporarily stop exercising. When you feel well enough to exercise again, don't try to pick up where you left off; instead, go back a step or two and gradually work up to your previous level. For example, if you had been working out for thirty or forty minutes at 75 percent of your maximum heart rate, try starting with ten or fifteen minutes at a lower level of intensity. After a few days, lengthen the workout and exercise a bit harder. You'll be pleasantly surprised to find how quickly you get back to your previous level.

Orthopedic problems. You may love running, but the high impact may be more than your ankles, knees, or back can tolerate. Check with an exercise physiologist, trainer, sports podiatrist, or physical therapist to see if your gait or shoes are responsible. If a change in shoes or corrective therapy doesn't help, you may need to switch to an activity that puts less stress on your joints. Swimming, stair stepping, cycling, or brisk walking may be more suitable and can provide an equally vigorous workout.

(*continued*)

(Box 5 *continued*)

Timing of workouts. Establish a regular routine when you can exercise at
   about the same time each day without feeling rushed. People's personali-
   ties are often divided into "morning" or "evening." Pick the time that
   works for you. Some like to exercise during the lunch break at work.
   (Avoid exercising shortly after eating, however; this can be harmful,
   especially if you have heart disease.) If you have difficulty sleeping,
   avoid vigorous exercise in the late evening. In contrast, stretching or
   weight training may help you relax and ease muscle tension at the
   end of the day.

every other day. During weeks two, three, four, and five, he increased his walking time by two minutes per session in each week (for example, twelve minutes
per session in week two, and fourteen minutes per session in week three), and
began walking twice a day four times a week.

Weeks six to nine began a cardiovascular conditioning phase for Stanley.
His exercise increased to a twenty-minute session five days a week. Resistance
training was introduced using free weights, starting with five-pound weights
and gradually working up to ten pounds. (Resistance exercise machines can be
used instead of free weights.) In weeks ten to thirteen, Stanley's exercise was increased to twenty-four minutes, five times a week, with the intensity gradually
increased to 60 percent of his maximum heart rate; he was given the option of
walking on a level surface, working out on a treadmill or exercise cycle, or water
aerobics (to accommodate his knee problems). During weeks fourteen to sixteen, Stanley continued to exercise for twenty-four minutes each session, but the
frequency was increased to six times a week. In weeks seventeen to nineteen, the
exercise was lengthened to twenty-eight minutes and its intensity was increased
to 65 percent of Stanley's maximum heart rate. He kept exercising for six sessions each week. In the final part of the conditioning phase, weeks twenty to
twenty-seven, Stanley was to work out for thirty minutes each session for six sessions a week. At the end of week twenty-seven, he was given a follow-up medical
checkup that included an ECG and exercise stress test. And starting in week
twenty-eight, he began a maintenance phase that continues today, in which he
sustains his exercise to forty minutes a session and continues to exercise five or
six times a week. He has been encouraged to vary his aerobic exercise to ease the
stress on his knees.

SUMMING UP

Age, other conditions, and initial cardiovascular health should not be barriers to starting an exercise program. Indeed, the right kinds of exercise can help counter common problems of aging or chronic disease. A groundbreaking study conducted in the late 1990s by Dr. Miriam E. Nelson (author of *Strong Women Stay Young*) of Tufts University documented the many benefits of weight training, along with aerobic exercise, in older women. Even women with advanced osteoporosis and severe arthritis experienced increased strength, improved balance, and even improved bone health, often after only a few weeks of starting an exercise program. Similarly, most people with heart disease, arthritis, asthma, or a host of other ailments also benefit from regular exercise. If you have health problems like these, it is important to plan your exercise program with your doctor, physical therapist, or other health professional trained to design regimens that meet special needs. Then you can safely join those who have already begun to achieve, through regular exercise, a stronger heart and healthier body.

3

Adopting a Heart-Healthy Diet

J̶ust as there is no successful one-size-fits-all exercise regimen, there is no single diet or nutrition program that works for everyone. The trick is to find a lifelong eating program that suits your taste while fitting in with your overall treatment goals. There is no doubt that the typical American diet—which is high in calories, saturated fats, red meats, cholesterol, potatoes and other starchy foods, sugar, and salt, and skimpy on vegetables, fruits, and whole grains—is a key factor in excessive weight gain. It also contributes to high blood pressure, high levels of blood cholesterol, and perhaps poor blood sugar control. Your genetic makeup is also a factor; if your parents and grandparents are overweight, chances are you will be too. Excess weight helps set the stage for atherosclerosis and heart disease, diabetes, high blood pressure, certain cancers, and a host of other diseases. In fact, obesity is now implicated in 300,000 American deaths a year, making it second only to cigarette smoking as a cause of preventable mortality.

To understand the magnitude of the problem, all you need to do is look around you (and perhaps in the mirror). In the United States alone, almost two-thirds of all adults are overweight or obese. Overweight is defined as having a body mass index (BMI) of 25 to 29.9, and any BMI over 30 is classified as obese (see Table 2 to determine your BMI.) The higher the BMI, the greater the risk of serious health problems and premature death, although there are conflicting data on where the risk begins. The ongoing Nurses' Health Study, conducted by investigators at Brigham and Women's Hospital in Boston, found that overweight participants suffered a higher death rate than their normal-weight counterparts, and the greater the weight, the higher the risk. In contrast, a 2005 report from the Centers for Disease Control found that being moderately overweight, with a BMI of 25 to 29.9, did not lead to premature death and, in fact, people in this range had a lower death rate than those who were markedly underweight (a BMI of less than 18.4). Statistics aside, there is no doubt that the health of far too many Americans suffers because of excess weight. Even more disconcerting is the increasing number of young children and adolescents who are overweight or obese.

The good news is that you can reduce your risk of heart disease and premature death by adopting a nutritionally sound, lifelong eating plan. The ideal plan, which also includes regular exercise, results in a gradual loss of excessive body fat and then the maintenance of a healthful weight. Success also results in enhanced self-esteem and stress reduction, whereas failure frequently produces opposite results.

While dieting sounds simple, for the vast majority of people, it's anything but. Take the case of Alice. When she had her heart attack at age forty-five, she was five feet, four inches tall and weighed 190 pounds, giving her a BMI of 33. In addition to being obese, Alice also had type II diabetes. Before suffering a major heart attack, she had tried a dozen or more diets—everything from peanut butter and liquid protein diets, to a strict low-fat scheme, to an egg and grapefruit plan. All of the diets produced pretty much the same results: "I'd lose a few pounds and feel pretty proud of myself," she recalls. "But before long, I couldn't stand feeling hungry and irritable all the time, and before I knew it, I was back in my old rut and whatever weight I'd lost would soon be right back where it was—mostly around my stomach."

When it came to providing specific dietary guidance, Alice's doctor wasn't much help. "He kept telling me to eat less and exercise more, and he sometimes gave me a printed diet," she recalls. "But hard as I tried, this just didn't work for me. I felt guilty and kept blaming myself for not having the willpower to stick to a workable plan."

Alice finally achieved success after having her heart attack and undergoing extensive counseling with a dietitian as part of her cardiac rehab program. For the first time, she realized that her previous failed attempts to lose weight were not due to a lack of willpower or moral strength. Instead, she simply had not worked out an eating program that was tailored to her individual needs and so could be sustained over the long haul. One important lesson Alice learned was that a diet that works well for one person may not produce the same results in

TABLE 2

BODY MASS INDEX

Body Mass Index (BMI) Table

BMI	19	20	21	22	23	24	25	26	27	28	29	30	31	32	33	34	35	40
Height							*Weight (in pounds)*											
4'10" (58")	91	96	100	105	110	115	119	124	129	134	138	143	148	153	158	162	167	191
4'11" (59")	94	99	104	109	114	119	124	128	133	138	143	148	153	158	163	168	173	198
5' (60")	97	102	107	112	118	123	128	133	138	143	148	153	158	163	168	174	179	204
5'1" (61")	100	106	111	116	122	127	132	137	143	148	153	158	164	169	174	180	185	211
5'2" (62")	104	109	115	120	126	131	136	142	147	153	158	164	169	175	180	186	191	218
5'3" (63")	107	113	118	124	130	135	141	146	152	158	163	169	175	180	186	191	197	225
5'4" (64")	110	116	122	128	134	140	145	151	157	163	169	174	180	186	192	197	204	232
5'5" (65")	114	120	126	132	138	144	150	156	162	168	174	180	186	192	198	204	210	240
5'6" (66")	118	124	130	136	142	148	155	161	167	173	179	186	192	198	204	210	216	247
5'7" (67")	121	127	134	140	146	153	159	166	172	178	185	191	198	204	211	217	223	255
5'8" (68")	125	131	138	144	151	158	164	171	177	184	190	197	203	210	216	223	230	262
5'9" (69")	128	135	142	149	155	162	169	176	182	189	196	203	209	216	223	230	236	270
5'10" (70")	132	139	146	153	160	167	174	181	188	195	202	209	216	222	229	236	243	278
5'11" (71")	136	143	150	157	165	172	179	186	193	200	208	215	222	229	236	243	250	286
6' (72")	140	147	154	162	169	177	184	191	199	206	213	221	228	235	242	250	258	294
6'1" (73")	144	151	159	166	174	182	189	197	204	212	219	227	235	242	250	257	265	302
6'2" (74")	148	155	163	171	179	186	194	202	210	218	225	233	241	249	256	264	272	311
6'3" (75")	152	160	168	176	184	192	200	208	216	224	232	240	248	256	264	272	279	319

How to interpret:

BMI	Classification
18.5 or less	Underweight
18.5–24.9	Normal Weight
25.0–29.9	Overweight
30.0–39.9	Obese
40 or greater	Very obese

Source: Centers for Disease Control and Prevention, U.S. Department of Health and Human Services, www.cdc.gov.

another, even though their individual circumstances may seem similar. The printed diets provided by her doctors were based on sound nutritional principles, but didn't work for Alice. Similarly, you should avoid blindly following a diet that works for a relative or friend without determining if it will work specifically for you.

Dr. Lisa Sanders emphasizes this point in her important book *The Perfect Fit Diet*. She notes that "anyone who has tried to diet knows that it's not about motivation. The key to being able to stay on a diet is how well that diet fits you as an individual." To find that elusive "perfect fit diet," one must start by recognizing that individual taste and food preferences must be considered. It's also important to understand that there are marked differences between people in the way they process or metabolize certain foods, such as starches and other carbohydrates. Dr. Sanders notes that "there is good evidence that small dissimilarities in several genes make dramatic differences in the ways some people respond to the amount and type of fat in their diets." In addition, Dr. Sanders reports that there are variations in what prompts people to feel full and stop eating, and that "what makes us stop eating is actually a very complicated process." In fact, studies of obese children found that some produce low levels of a brain hormone that prompts a feeling of satiety. Dr. Sanders writes: "The clear implication is that these children may be obese simply because they never really feel full or satisfied by a meal."

Personality is also a factor. For a methodical person who likes to keep records, a diet that emphasizes counting calories, fats, carbohydrates, and so on may be appropriate. For others, a broad plan that allows ample food choices and substitutions may work better.

A COMMONSENSE APPROACH TO DIETING

Alice's experience is an all-too-common example of why so many diets fail. "I'd go on one for a few weeks, and then fall off," she recounts. If you have a weight problem, chances are that you too have vowed to go on a diet, perhaps selecting the one that hit the best-seller list this year. This is where so many people make what we consider their big mistake in trying to control their weight: trying a one-size-fits-all approach rather than taking into account individual differences and needs. Typically, the person tries such a diet for a while, and like Alice, may enjoy initial success. But if he or she then reverts to former eating habits, rather than instituting permanent change, the lost weight will soon return. So instead of starting your diet by buying the latest diet book, carefully analyze what and how you eat. Alice's dietitian instructed her to keep a daily diary of everything she ate for a week, including the time of day and circumstances. (It's important to make the diary entries when you eat rather than try to reconstruct the day's food intake hours later.) The dietitian also asked Alice to list her favorite foods and describe why she liked each. Was it the sweet taste? Texture? Convenience or ease of preparation? She also instructed her to list some foods she didn't like or seldom ate, and again, to explain why. Did the foods fail to satisfy her hunger? Were they too bitter or sour? Too expensive? Hard to find or prepare? Too unfamiliar?

The dietitian then sat down with Alice to analyze her diet and list of food preferences. Alice tended to snack a lot, usually on potato chips, cheese and crackers, nuts, and other calorie-dense foods. Her meals invariably included a meat, poultry, or fish dish; bread; and potatoes or another starch. Only occasionally did she include a vegetable or salad. She drank a lot of coffee, fruit juice, and diet soft drinks, but not much water or milk. Because of her diabetes, she avoided sugary desserts, but confessed to a fondness for chocolate.

Using this information, the dietitian recommended a nutritious eating plan that Alice could adopt as part of her lifelong health program. In Alice's case, the plan was based on Dr. Arthur Agatston's popular *South Beach Diet*. It allowed frequent snacks, although not the fatty ones that Alice had preferred. Still, the frequent small snacks helped prevent the gnawing hunger that had doomed Alice's earlier efforts. The meal plans provided ample low-fat, high-protein entrees, but with more emphasis on vegetables and green salads than provided in Alice's normal menus. Although it did not include some of Alice's favorite foods, such as bread, pasta, and potatoes, her dietitian was able to suggest modifications, such as occasional servings of whole-grain pasta and bread, that were in keeping with her health needs and taste. Perhaps best of all, this particular diet allowed a daily "dose" of low-sugar dark chocolate in various forms. Alice found the recipes simple and fast to prepare—important considerations given her busy schedule. With sensible modifications, this particular diet came close to fitting Alice's food preferences while helping her lose weight and control her blood sugar.

Of course, what worked for Alice may not necessarily be the right choice for you. Find a similar structured approach that is likely to work for your situation. You may want to start by consulting a dietitian or a doctor with an interest in nutrition. A word of caution, however: be wary of a nutrition counselor who suggests a rigid diet without first determining what you eat, what foods you like, and your circumstances. (For example: Do you eat most of your meals at home or in restaurants? When do you do most of your eating? Do you sit down for family meals or eat on the run?) It's also a good idea to make this a family affair, especially

Box 6

TEN TIPS FOR CONTROLLING YOUR DIET

People who are overweight tend to share certain food preferences and eating habits. Identifying and then modifying these greatly increase your chances of successful weight loss. Start by going through the following questions and tips for making small but very important changes.

1. When I'm hungry, I crave (a) sweets, (b) cheese and other high-fat foods, (c) crackers, bread, and other starchy foods, (d) potato chips, salted nuts, and other salty foods, or (e) other.

    Tips for change: If you crave sweets, look for sugar-free foods that satisfy your cravings but are low in calories and refined carbohydrates; examples include low-fat sugar-free ice cream or yogurt; an apple, pear, berries, or other nontropical fruits; and sugar-free ginger snaps or similar cookies. An ounce or so of low-sugar dark chocolate also satisfies a sweet tooth and has some real health benefits, including lowering blood pressure and improving vascular function.

2. I want each meal to include (a) a meat dish, (b) potatoes or another starchy food, or (c) rich dessert.

    Tips for change: Emphasize lean meats, fish, or poultry over steaks, burgers, chops, and other high-fat, high-calorie choices. Instead of potatoes, pasta, and white rice, substitute a whole-grain, high-fiber dish such as kasha, brown rice, or whole-wheat couscous. Instead of a pastry or other high-sugar, high-fat dessert, try a baked apple (flavored with cinnamon instead of loads of sugar) topped with a spoonful of low-fat sugar-free ice cream.

3. On a typical day, I have _____ servings of fruits and vegetables.

    Tips for change: Strive for at least eight or nine servings—the amount now recommended in the new Food Guide Pyramid. While this may sound like a lot, it's relatively easy to get if you have many salads, at least one or two vegetables at each meal, and snack on fruit or raw veggies instead of high-fat or sugary foods.

4. Yes or no: I regularly skip breakfast.

    Tips for change: There's a lot of truth to the old saw popularized by Jane Brody, the *New York Times* personal health columnist: "Eat a breakfast for a king, a lunch for a prince, and dinner for a pauper." Skipping breakfast means that by midmorning you're likely to feel very hungry and overeat. And if you also skimp on lunch, by dinnertime your body will be

(continued)

(Box 6 *continued*)

in desperate need of food, and you're likely to consume many more calories than you ordinarily would if you'd eaten during the day.

5. Yes or no: I always feel compelled to eat everything on my plate, whether I'm hungry or not.

   Tips for change: Forget what your mother said about always cleaning your plate. Take small portions and stop eating when you no longer feel hungry. If you can't bear to toss the leftovers, save them for a later snack or another meal.

6. Yes or no: I'm invariably the first person to finish a meal.

   Tips for change: Make a conscious effort to slow down. People who tend to wolf down their food invariably eat more than they need to satisfy their hunger. Chew each mouthful slowly, put down your fork between bites, engage in conversation with your dining companions. By eating more slowly, you give your appetite control center a chance to signal your brain that you've had enough.

7. When I'm thirsty, I'm most likely to reach for (a) a soda or other soft drink, (b) fruit juice, (c) coffee or tea, (d) a beer, or (e) water.

   Tips for change: As a rule, you should consume the equivalent of six glasses of fluids a day, and your choices can really add the calories. Regular sodas and fruit juice are high in calories; so too are beer and other alcoholic beverages. Water, sugar-free soft drinks, or a cup or two of coffee or tea (sweetened as desired with a sugar substitute) satisfy thirst and don't add unwanted calories.

8. Yes or no: I usually snack while watching TV or when relaxing.

   Tips for change: Snacking while watching TV is a common habit, and one that can add the calories if you turn to chips, cookies, nuts, candy, and similar munchies. If you must eat in front of the TV, try unbuttered popcorn (check the label for fat and calorie counts), a piece of fruit or raw veggies (a good way to reach your servings goal), or a few whole-grain crackers.

9. Yes or no: When food shopping, I always read the labels.

   Tips for change: Congratulations if you answered "yes." If you don't read labels, get in the habit of doing so. You'll quickly be able to identify foods that are high in nutrition and low in sugar, fats, and calories. You can also spot harmful ingredients, such as trans fats (the artificially hardened fats found in many margarines and processed foods) or tropical oils (palm, palm kernel, and coconut oils).

10. Yes or no: When I go through a cafeteria line, I load my plate with everything that's offered, and then eat it all.

Tips for change: If you answered "yes" to this question, you're by no means alone. All those dishes can be very tempting. Take a small plate and pick one or two selections; eat those slowly, and then if you're still hungry, go back for another sample or two.

By now, you get the picture. Take the time to analyze your food preferences and eating habits; you'll soon be able to spot those that are contributing to your weight problem and make the minor adjustments that can make a big difference.

if you do not do the food shopping and preparation. In any event, keep track of everything you eat for at least a week, and then study this diary for clues about habits that merit modifying (see Box 6, Ten Tips for Controlling Your Diet).

Just as your exercise regimen should be a lifelong program, so too should be your nutrition plan. Let flexibility and common sense dictate your diet-for-life plan. Far too many people regard a diet as temporary—a strategy to follow only until a goal is achieved (lose a few or many pounds, bring blood sugar under control, and so on)—and then revert to their former unhealthy way of eating. This approach typically leads to yo-yo dieting, rather than a healthful, lifelong eating program. This doesn't mean you can't occasionally indulge in a treat that's not part of your eating plan. Enjoy and then get back on the program! Remember, this is a lifelong endeavor, and one that should accommodate your individual likes and dislikes as well as meet your specific health needs. If you accept this diet-for-life concept, there are no permanent setbacks and no permanent failures—you can partake in a special holiday meal or take a vacation from your diet when you really need to. Afterward, simply return to your eating plan and take up where you left off. This is what Alice did during the Christmas and New Year's holidays. "I decided I was going to enjoy a few days of my favorite dishes, and not even step on the scale," she recalls. "I knew that I had gone a bit too far when I had trouble fitting into my new smaller size jeans. So I just went back to the weight-loss phase, and when I had shed the five pounds I gained over the holidays, I again advanced to the maintenance program."

Understandably, most people with a weight problem long for a magic pill or potion that will melt off unwanted pounds effortlessly. Despite all those seductive TV commercials and magazine articles and ads, such a magic bullet simply does not exist. The medical literature is full of accounts of weight-loss drugs and supplements that created more problems than they solved. In fact some, such as Fen-phen (Phentermine and Fenfluramine), Pondimin, and Redux, proved to have very significant medical complications. Amphetamines and nutrition supplements with amphetamine-like compounds have caused addiction and serious, even fatal, heart problems. Be wary of any product, be it a prescription drug or over-the-counter remedy, that promises rapid weight loss without your having to change the way you eat.

SURGICAL TREATMENTS

Another treatment strategy currently in vogue involves bariatric surgery to either reduce stomach size or bypass parts of the stomach or small intestine to reduce the amount of food that can be consumed and absorbed. This approach has been boosted by testimonials from a number of overweight celebrities who have slimmed down after having the surgery. A case in point is Deborah Voigt, the opera singer. She made headlines in 2004 when London's Royal Opera canceled her contract to sing Ariadne auf Naxos—one of her signature roles—because she couldn't fit into the black cocktail dress the production manager and costume designer had selected. She again made the news in 2005 when the *New York Times* featured on the front page a photo of a slim Ms. Voigt wearing a size fourteen black dress, and revealed that she had lost at least a hundred pounds after undergoing bariatric surgery several months earlier.

The American Society for Bariatric Surgery (ASBS) recommends that these operations be limited to patients who are morbidly obese—that is, with a BMI of forty or more and at least one hundred pounds overweight—and unable to lose weight through less drastic means. Several types of operations are available, but most entail reducing the size of the stomach. The most common of the surgeries involve using staples or special bands to reduce the stomach's size and create a pouch that holds only a limited amount of food. The smaller stomach forces patients to consume small amounts of food at any given time, to eat slowly, and to chew the food thoroughly. Overeating or eating too fast can result in vomiting.

In some procedures, a portion of the small intestine is also tied off. This type of intestinal bypass surgery reduces the amount of food that is absorbed into the body, and to prevent nutritional deficiencies, patients often need to take dietary supplements. Regardless of the type of operation, the maximum weight loss usually occurs within eighteen months to two years after surgery. Long-term follow-up studies show that, despite losing half or more of their preoperative weight, about half of patients still do not achieve normal weight (a BMI of less than twenty-five). But they do benefit from improvement in many obesity-related disorders—including type II diabetes, sleep apnea, and high blood pressure— as well as enhanced cardiovascular function, self-esteem, and quality of life. Even so, bariatric surgery should not be attempted without careful consideration of possible adverse effects. According to the ASBS, about 10 percent of patients suffer potentially serious side effects, which include infection, a breakdown of the stomach staples resulting in leakage, the formation of dangerous blood clots in the legs (deep venous thrombophlebitis), ulcers, and nutritional problems. Some patients experience digestive problems, including frequent heartburn and chronic diarrhea or constipation. Although these complications can usually be managed by careful attention to diet and eating habits, such as frequent small meals, in some patients they are severe enough to require reversal of the surgery.

DIETS: DIFFERENT APPROACHES TO WEIGHT LOSS

Although most weight-loss diets stress a particular point of view—counting calories, restricting fat or carbohydrates, or limiting food selection, among others—in order to work, they must induce you to take in less energy than you expend. This is the only way that you can shed unwanted pounds.

Counting Calories

No matter how you cut it, calories do count, and every weight-loss diet—low- or high-fat, low- or high-carbohydrate, low- or high-protein—reduces caloric intake. Although metabolism varies depending on your genetic makeup and other individual factors, if you eat more calories than you burn, the excess will be converted to fat and stored for future use. The problem is, most of us do not call on these reserves, but continue overeating, underexercising, and piling on the pounds. In general, 3,500 unburned calories turns into a pound of body fat. (To take in 3,500 calories in a single meal [give or take a few calories depending on serving size], you can consume a double cheeseburger, large order of french fries, a half-liter of cola, side of coleslaw, a triple-scoop ice cream cone with chopped nuts, and a super-size chocolate chip cookie.)

Conversely, if you burn more calories than you take in, you'll gradually lose weight. For example, you can theoretically lose a pound by walking five miles every day for a week, provided you do not change your food intake. Of course, not everyone can walk this far. So obviously, the best approach is one that combines a moderate reduction in calories with an increase in exercise, which not only burns calories but also helps curb appetite.

While cutting calories and increasing exercise—even in modest amounts—help control weight, incorporating these changes into your lifestyle is not as simple as it sounds. For one thing, any drastic reduction in calories prompts the body to respond by slowing metabolism to conserve energy. This is a defensive mechanism that dates to the early feast-or-famine days of human evolution. During times of plenty, the body stored unused energy as fat. During lean times, metabolism slowed down to stave off starvation. Today, lean times are rare in developed nations, but we still eat as if a famine may come tomorrow. Ergo the current obesity epidemic. Any successful weight-loss plan calls for a gradual loss of weight without slowing metabolism—something that can be accomplished by increasing exercise and at the same time reducing food consumption to 1,000 to 1,500 calories a day (compared to the 2,500 to 3,500 or more calories in the typical American diet). This combination of exercising and consuming enough food prevents the starvation "slow-down." Accomplishing your weight-loss goal, then, will require not only exercise, but also carefully selecting low-calorie foods that are high in nutrition, moderating portion size, and developing a lifelong eating plan that takes into account your food preferences and individual nutritional needs.

As noted by Dr. Sanders: "The trick to any successful diet is to eat fewer calories but to do it in a way that fools your body and brain into feeling that you are satisfied and never hungry." This may mean increasing intake of whole-grain products, along with small amounts of olive oil or other unsaturated fats, which are digested slowly and give a feeling of fullness. Or you can eat more low-calorie, high-fiber vegetables. In general, calorie-counter diets call for a balance of high-fiber carbohydrates, low-fat protein, and a moderate amount of fat (preferably poly- or monounsaturated fats like olive, canola, or walnut oils). This type of diet works best for people disciplined enough to keep an accurate food diary and to use tables to calculate the numbers of calories in each serving. Portion control is emphasized; common examples include diets offered by Weight Watchers and Jenny Craig.

Cutting Fats

Fat contains more calories (nine per gram) than protein or carbohydrates (four per gram), so it's logical that many popular diets drastically reduce fat intake.

Be careful, however, because many "lite" or low-fat foods replace fat with increased sugar, so they may have just as many calories as their high-fat counterparts. Other foods, such as low- or no-fat cheese, are loaded with extra salt to make them palatable and may not be suitable for people with high blood pressure. Remember, too, that controlling portion size is critical. Many people think that if a food is labeled "lite," "low-fat," or "sugar-free" they can eat all they want without suffering adverse consequences. Yet although one or two heart-healthy cookies are fine, eating the whole package at a sitting is anything but heart healthy.

The typical low-fat diet restricts fat intake to 10 to 20 percent of total calories, compared to 40 percent or more in the typical American diet. Because fat promotes satiety by slowing digestion and metabolism, adds flavor, and gives food a pleasing texture, many low- or fat-free foods are bland and may not curb hunger for an extended period. Low-fat diets are best suited to people who enjoy a mostly vegetarian fare—for example, lots of pasta, veggies, fruits, whole grains, and beans. Examples of low-fat diets are those developed by Dr. Dean Ornish (*Eat More, Weigh Less*) and Dr. Neal Barnard (*Turn Off the Fat Genes*). Although experts disagree, in general very fat-restricted diets (10 to 20 percent of calories) may not be recommended for persons with diabetes, metabolic syndrome, or low levels of HDL (good) cholesterol. The American Heart Association diet allows more fat—up to 30 percent of calories—and some Weight Watchers diets allow a similar amount of fat.

Not all fats are equal when it comes to heart health. Numerous studies show that saturated fats—those found in most red meats, tropical oils, and dairy products, as well as those that have been artificially saturated to remain hard at room temperature—promote atherosclerosis by interfering with the removal of LDL (bad) cholesterol from the blood. Saturated fats are also a precursor to cholesterol and have a greater effect on raising blood cholesterol than dietary cholesterol itself. In contrast, mono- and polyunsaturated fats, which come from plant sources and are liquid at room temperature, help lower blood cholesterol. In this regard, polyunsaturates—the oils from cottonseed, sunflowers, safflower, soybeans, corn, and nuts—are the more beneficial because they appear to lower LDL, although they can also reduce HDL. Monounsaturates, which are found in canola, olive, peanut, and cashew oils, also help lower cholesterol.

Body fat is also important in the metabolism of cholesterol. In particular, fat in the abdominal area is more metabolically active than fat stored elsewhere in the body, which is why excessive abdominal fat raises the risk of heart disease.

Counting Carbs

Low-carbohydrate diets are among the newest weight-loss plans, and in the last decade or so, they have gained a following among people who want to lose weight. In general, low-carb diets turn the traditional food pyramid on its head. Instead of getting 60 percent or more of calories from starches and other carbohydrates, only about 20 percent come from this food group, with the bulk of calories coming from protein and fat.

The Atkins diet, one of the oldest and most popular of the low-carb plans, stresses meat, fish, poultry, eggs, dairy products, nuts, fats, and oils, while eliminating or restricting fruits, potatoes and other starchy foods, and sugar, at least during the initial phases. (In the maintenance phase, salads, high-fiber vegetables, and some fruits are included.) A newer, more moderate approach is outlined in Dr. Arthur Agatston's *South Beach Diet,* which puts more emphasis on low-fat protein sources and allows more low-starch vegetables than does the Atkins diet. Both diets restrict or eliminate sugar and refined starchy foods (for example, white bread, bagels, regular pasta, and white rice), which are quickly metabolized to blood sugar. This sugar prompts the body to release insulin, the hormone instrumental in carbohydrate metabolism. Surges in insulin are also said to promote fat storage, another reason why sugar and starches are restricted in low-carb diets.

Although experts disagree on the merits of low-carb diets, there is little doubt that they can result in substantial weight loss without promoting hunger. At first glance, it would seem that a diet such as that developed by Dr. Atkins, which sets no limits on steaks, lobster, butter, bacon, cheese, and other such foods, would promote weight gain rather than loss. And indeed, some people do gain weight on this type of diet. But many who faithfully follow a high-protein, high-fat, low-carbohydrate diet shed pounds. They also report increased energy, and may even enjoy lowered blood cholesterol and improved blood sugar control. How can this be? When carefully analyzed, these diets reduce total caloric intake even while allowing all sorts of fatty, calorie-dense foods. After all, how much lobster, bacon, or steak can you eat without feeling full? Such diets also reduce surges in insulin, which may slow fat storage.

It is not fully understood how these high-fat, high-protein diets lower blood cholesterol, but studies show that many, although not all, people following these regimens achieve this objective. The Atkins diet, high in fats and cholesterol, would also be expected to raise blood cholesterol levels, which happens in some people. But for reasons that are not yet understood, some people enjoy the opposite effect, and their cholesterol levels actually fall on the diet. This is just another example of the need to tailor any diet or eating plan to the individual.

In any event, low-carb diets seem to work best for people who like lots of meat, poultry, fish, and other high-protein foods, and don't miss pasta, potatoes, and cereals, breads, and baked goods made with refined flours. Note too that these diets are staged, so that after you progress past the first few weeks of restricted foods, during which many people lose ten or more pounds and may also normalize blood sugar, you can start adding back moderate amounts of grains, beans, and other high-fiber carbohydrates. (Table 3 compares some of the more popular weight-loss diets.)

Using the 2005 Food Guide Pyramid

The government's 2005 version of the Food Guide Pyramid is designed to reduce calories and increase exercise. Unlike the previous pyramid, which allowed eleven servings of grains and starches a day, the new pyramid shifts the emphasis to vegetables and fruits—foods that are lower in calories and higher in vitamins and minerals than most starches. It calls for nine servings a day of these foods. A serving is defined as a half cup of cooked vegetables or fruits or a cup of raw foods. The new pyramid also urges at least thirty minutes of exercise a day—a recommendation that was not included in previous versions. (Table 4 provides an overview of the pyramid for different population groups.)

Regional and Ethnic Diets

Numerous population studies document the benefits of certain ethnic diets. High on the list is the traditional Mediterranean diet, which emphasizes complex carbohydrates (grains, beans, vegetables), starches (pasta and rice), fish, and olives and olive oil, with moderate amounts of meats and sweets. A European study, published in 2004 in the *Journal of the American Medical Association* (*JAMA*), followed more than 2,300 elderly subjects, aged seventy to ninety years, in nineteen European centers for up to ten years. In this study, those elderly persons who consumed a Mediterranean diet, consumed alcohol in moderation, abstained from smoking, and exercised regularly had a 50 percent lower death rate when compared to counterparts who did not follow this diet and lifestyle.

The traditional Asian diet, which emphasizes vegetables, fruits, fiber, rice, and mono- or polyunsaturated oils and is low in meat and sweets, has also been linked to increased longevity and a reduced risk of heart disease. Similar benefits

TABLE 3

POPULAR DIETS COMPARED

Type/Example	Basics	Pros	Cons
Very low-fat/ Dr. Ornish's *Eat More, Weigh Less*	Limits fat intake to 10 percent of total calories; emphasizes grains, vegetables, fruits; limits or eliminates many meats, dairy products, and other such foods	Has been shown to lower blood cholesterol, improve diabetes control, and cause weight loss; may slow or even reverse buildup of fatty plaque in the arteries.	Difficult to follow for any length of time; many people complain of a lack of flavor and texture consistent with diets that provide more fat.
Calorie-counter diets/Weight Watchers; American Heart Association	Limit fat to 30 to 35 percent of calories; stress moderate portion size.	Diets provide for gradual weight loss; they allow a wide variety of foods and can be adapted to suit individual tastes.	Few drawbacks, although some people have difficulty following plans for the long haul and regain lost weight as they slip back into former eating habits.
High-protein, low-carb diets/ Dr. Atkins's *Diet Revolution;* Dr. Sears's *The Zone*	Carbohydrate intake restricted to 20 to 30 percent of calories; sugar, refined grain products, potatoes, and other starches are restricted.	Diets best suited to people who crave a lot of meats and other high-protein foods. Adherents do not feel hungry and many lose weight quickly.	High intake of fats and high-protein foods may harm kidneys and may raise cholesterol in some people; many highly nutritious foods are restricted.
Low-carb, low-glycemic diets/ Dr. Agatston's *South Beach Diet*	Restricts starchy foods, sugar, fruit, refined flours, and carbohydrates; emphasizes low-fat sources of protein; allows many vegetables.	Diet produces gradual weight loss; helps control blood sugar. Frequent snacks help prevent hunger; after initial phases, diet is varied enough to satisfy most tastes.	Initial phases require considerable discipline.

TABLE 4

HOW TO USE THE 2005 FOOD GUIDE PYRAMID

Food group	Amount in 2000-calorie diet	Daily servings for women	Daily servings for men	Daily servings for children over age four
Grains (half from whole grains)	6 ounces (e.g. 4–5 servings)	6 ounces	8 ounces (5–6 servings)	5 ounces (3–4 servings)
Vegetables	2½ cups (5 servings)	2½ cups (5 servings)	3 cups (6 servings)	1½ cups (3 one-half cup servings; 6 quarter-cup servings)
Fruits	2 cups (4 servings)	2 cups (4 servings)	3 cups (6 servings)	2 cups (4 servings)
Milk (low-fat)	3 cups	3 cups	3 cups	2 cups
Meat/beans	5½ ounces	5 ounces	6 ounces	3–4 ounces
Fats and sweets	Limit	Limit	Limit	Limit

Source: U.S. Department of Agriculture.

have been attributed to vegetarian diets as well as other ethnic diets that are high in fiber, vegetables, fruits, and oils, but low in saturated fats, red meats, and sugar.

THE BENEFITS OF WINE

Much has been written in recent years about the benefits of wine, especially red wine, for the heart. (Similar benefits have been linked to moderate consumption of brandy, spirits, and other alcoholic drinks.) This is sometimes referred to as the "French factor" because the French generally enjoy a low risk of heart disease despite their consumption of large amounts of rich sauces, cheese, and other fatty foods. The French fondness for wine has been cited as a possible explanation. Of course, the benefits are not limited to the French. In the United States, a long-term study of some 38,000 male health professionals found that those who consumed moderate amounts of wine (one to three glasses on most days of the week) enjoyed a reduced risk of heart disease when compared to teetotalers. This is attributed, in part, to the fact that moderate wine consumption can raise levels of HDL (good) cholesterol, even though the precise protective substance in wine is unknown. Some experts theorize that substances called phytochemicals, especially the kind found in purple grape skins, protect against heart disease.

Importantly, while moderate wine consumption may be beneficial, there are some people, such as those with chronic liver disease or persons taking medications that interact with alcohol, who should not consume any alcohol. Excessive alcohol consumption can also harm rather than benefit the heart. Remember, too, that alcohol is high in calories—about seven calories per gram. This translates to about 120 calories in a six-ounce glass of wine (11.5 percent alcohol), 145 calories in twelve ounces of beer (4.5 percent alcohol), and about 100 calories for 1.5 ounces of 86-proof gin, rum, vodka, or whiskey. For people who can't drink or choose not to, some of the antioxidants and phytochemicals in red wine can be obtained by drinking purple grape juice. Be careful, however, because grape juice tends to be high in sugar.

A PINCH OF SALT

Table salt, or sodium chloride, is an electrolyte, a component essential for maintaining the body's proper fluid and chemical balance. It raises blood pressure in susceptible persons, especially those of African descent. According to the American Heart Association (AHA), the average American consumes at least twice as much salt a day than is considered healthy. Everyone can benefit from moderating their salt intake, but it is especially important for people who have high blood pressure and/or congestive heart failure to do so. The AHA recommends that persons with high blood pressure cut their salt intake to about 600 milligrams, or about a quarter teaspoonful, a day. (Some people may find this level of restriction unpalatable; if so, talk to your doctor or dietitian about possibly allowing more.) This means reading labels for sodium content and eliminating most processed foods from the diet. Alternative flavorings, such as pepper, cinnamon, garlic, and lemon juice, can be used instead. (Table 5 lists the sodium content of common foods.)

Tips to Lower Your Salt Intake

The average American diet contains six to eighteen grams of salt, or one to three teaspoonfuls, a day. People on a salt-restricted diet should limit intake to six hundred milligrams, about one-fourth of a teaspoon, which is still more than

TABLE 5

SALT CONTENT IN COMMON FOODS

Food/Portion Size	Sodium Content (average milligrams)
Meats	
Canadian-style bacon/2 slices (1.5 ounces)	710
Ham/3 ounces	900
Frankfurter/1 medium	500–800
Salami/1 ounce	300
Fish and Shellfish	
Lox/1 ounce	570
Canned tuna/3 ounces	320
Canned salmon/3 ounces	470
Canned sardines/3 ounces	425
Steamed mussels/3 ounces	570
Canned Soups	
Bean with bacon/1 cup	950
Chicken noodle/1 cup	950
Minestrone/1 cup	910
Tomato/1 cup	870
Mushroom/1 cup	1,030
Chicken bouillon/1 cube	1,150
Dairy Products	
American cheese/1 ounce	405
Blue cheese/1 ounce	400
Parmesan/1 ounce ungrated	530
Low-fat cottage cheese/1/2 cup	460
Butter, regular/1 tablespoon	115
Milk, regular or low-fat/1 cup	120
Yogurt, plain low-fat/1 cup	160
Snack Foods	
Salted mixed nuts/1 ounce	185
Salted dry-roasted peanuts/1 ounce	120
Peanut butter/1 tablespoon	75
Dill pickle/1 medium	930
Pretzels/1 ounce	475
Potato chips/1 ounce	130
Corn chips/1 ounce	235
Instant chocolate pudding	440

Note: *This is a very abbreviated list; check the food labels for the sodium content of prepared or convenience foods and select those that are low in salt, preferably less than 200 milligrams per serving.*

Source: Adapted from Victor Herbert, M.D., and Genell Subak-Sharpe, *Total Nutrition: The Only Guide You'll Ever Need* (New York: St. Martin's Press, 1995).

the two hundred milligrams a day that the body needs. Here are some suggestions from the American Heart Association:

- ♥ Remove the salt shaker from the table; use pepper and other flavorings instead.
- ♥ Never salt food before tasting it, an all-too-common habit.
- ♥ Don't use added salt during cooking; try herbs, spices, lemon juice, or a salt-free flavoring mix instead.
- ♥ Check food labels for salt (sodium) content, and select those that are low-salt.
- ♥ Cut back on salty snack foods; try spicy (unsalted) popcorn, raw vegetables or fruits, unsalted nuts or seeds, among others.
- ♥ Cut back on canned or processed foods, which tend to be high in added salt; look for brands that are labeled low-salt.
- ♥ Switch to low-salt or unsalted butter and condiments. Mustard, mayonnaise, catsup, relish, and other condiments are usually very high in salt.
- ♥ Don't be fooled by taste; many foods that taste sweet are actually very high in salt.
- ♥ When dining out, ask that your food be prepared without salt. (Some ethnic foods, especially those offered in Chinese and other Asian restaurants, tend to be very high in salt, but most restaurants will offer low-salt alternatives.)

SUMMING UP

Diet is not a sometimes thing—it's what you eat and drink every day of your life. If you are overweight or have a nutrition-related health disorder, you will probably have to alter your eating habits until the problem is under control. But these changes should be part of your lifelong eating, exercise, and treatment plan. Yo-yo dieting is not the answer; in fact, it can make matters worse by altering metabolism and promoting accelerated weight gain. As Alice, a patient featured in this chapter, learned, developing a diet that may work for you and adjusting the diet as needed can lead to long-term success. For most people, a healthy diet will include moderate portion size and added variety in the form of high-fiber whole grains, vegetables, and low-fat protein sources, among other nutritious food choices. When coupled with regular exercise and attention to the other lifestyle factors discussed in this book, a heart-healthy diet can be an important step toward your lifelong wellness.

4

Stress, Depression, and Other Psychological Factors

Practicing physicians and researchers alike have long observed that a sizable percentage of heart attack patients are apparently free of the accepted risk factors, such as high blood pressure, elevated blood cholesterol, and tobacco use. Why do these seemingly healthy, low-risk persons fall victim to a heart attack? A number of studies conducted in the last two decades suggest that psychological factors may play an important role.

We are not trained psychologists, so although much of what we discuss here is based on our experience treating patients and observing family interactions, we cannot offer professional advice on how to treat any psychological disorder. Moreover, although an impressive body of evidence has been amassed linking psychological factors and heart disease, this relationship remains an area of continuing debate. Still, the significance of psychological factors and personality cannot be ignored. Certainly persons who are under constant stress or suffering from depression, anxiety, and certain other psychological problems should do whatever they can to minimize detrimental effects on overall health and the heart in particular.

WHAT IS STRESS?

There is no single definition of stress, but it is generally agreed that stress involves both physical and psychological components. We all encounter various degrees of stress in our daily lives—for example, standing in line at the post office or supermarket, arguing with a family member or colleague, rushing to meet a deadline or appointment. Obviously, some stressors, such as the death of a loved one, loss of a job, divorce, or being caught up in a natural disaster, are more likely to have a severe impact on health than milder, positive stressors such as a job promotion or a child's achievement. Many heart attacks occur on the heels of particularly stressful episodes, both negative and positive. In addition, it is well documented that the death of a spouse is often followed by the death of the survivor within a short period of time. We often hear people refer to this as "dying of a broken heart."

There is much we have yet to learn about the complex brain-body interaction. But it is well documented that stress and excessive anger perceived in certain parts of the brain lead to complex hormonal changes. In turn, these hormonal changes can have a very profound influence on cardiovascular function, blood pressure, heart rate, circulation, and the ECG. There is also a growing body of evidence that stress affects the immune system—we are more susceptible to colds and other illnesses during periods of stress. Stress also appears to play a significant role in the health of patients with other classic risk factors and/or diagnosed heart disease. To bolster this contention, thousands of interviews with heart attack patients have pinpointed common traits, behavioral responses, and stress reactions that may increase their cardiovascular risk.

It's impossible to remove all stress from one's life; indeed, a certain amount of stress is desirable and is an integral part of many pleasurable and worthwhile activities. Dr. Hans Selye, a pioneer stress researcher of the 1930s, coined the word "eustress" to describe beneficial stress as opposed to detrimental "distress." In general, eustress is associated with exhilaration, happiness, or the feeling of a job well done. In contrast, distress leaves you feeling angry, anxious, tired, or simply out-of-sorts. (See Box 7 for a summary of indicators of stress.)

Regardless of the source of the stress, it triggers an automatic reaction, commonly referred to as the "fight-or-flight response." When faced with a stressful situation, the body's defensive mechanisms instantly go into action. Stress prompts the pituitary and adrenal glands to release stimulatory hormones, which ready the body to fight or flee. The heartbeat quickens, blood pressure rises, and blood rushes to the large muscles and brain. These responses can set the stage for increased strain on the heart and result in relatively reduced blood flow to the heart muscle (myocardial ischemia), a cause of angina. In laboratory settings, causing stress produces significant abnormalities in heart function, including reduced blood flow to the heart muscle in patients with known coronary artery disease.

Box 7

INDICATORS OF STRESS

Physical Signs

Facial tautness
Muscle tension, aches, or stiffness
Profuse sweating or flushing
Cold, clammy hands
Facial tics such as rapid eye blinking
Tapping foot or drumming fingers
Headaches
Sleep problems
Dizziness
Intestinal symptoms such as nausea, stomachache, diarrhea, or constipation
Fatigue
Skin rashes or hives
Back pain
Breathing problems (inability to get enough air to take a deep breath)
Dry mouth or throat
Palpitations and possible chest pains
Change in appetite

Emotional Indicators

Anger
Feelings of frustration
Withdrawal or lack of emotional feeling
Excessive crying without an obvious cause
Feelings of depression
Anxiety
Panic attack, fears, or phobias
Irritability and impatience
Forgetfulness or feelings of confusion
Difficulty concentrating
Feeling rushed or under time pressure

Behavioral Indicators

Rapid speech
Alcohol abuse

(*continued*)

(Box 7 *continued*)

Teeth grinding
Chain smoking
Restlessness or inability to sit or stand still
Nail-biting or picking at skin around nails or on the face
Hair-twisting
Impulsive eating
Sexual problems

Source: Adapted from B. L. Zaret, M. Moser, and L. S. Cohen, eds., *Yale University School of Medicine Heart Book* (New York: Hearst Books, 1992).

FAMILY DYNAMICS

Many studies have found that heart patients who have a strong emotional support system do better than those who live alone or lack support. Alternatively, stress can take a toll not only on the patient under stress, but also on family members and close friends. Stanley, the fifty-five-year-old executive, is a case in point. He readily admits that his unrelenting work schedule led to undue stress both at home and on the road. Stanley's wife, Marilyn, resented being left alone with their two teenage children for several days each week, and when her husband was home, he never had the time or energy (or perhaps desire) to participate in family activities. She felt angry that Stanley often forgot to take his heart medication, and she often nagged him about his lack of exercise and poor dietary habits. Understandably, this led to a lot of tension and resentment for both individuals.

After Stanley's heart attack and bypass surgery, his wife was determined to take charge and make sure that her husband did, indeed, turn over a new leaf. She accompanied him to his cardiac rehab sessions, and met with both his doctor and dietitian. "Before I knew it, I was a harping nag," she now admits. Despite her well-meaning efforts, within a few months Stanley had reverted to many of his old unhealthful ways, and Marilyn was more resentful, angry, and frustrated than ever. She feared that her husband would have another, perhaps fatal heart attack unless she took control and forced him to change. And although Stanley felt guilty, he resented Marilyn's approach.

This is an all-too-common scenario, and one that has no simple or universal solution. How can a concerned spouse or partner be supportive and nurturing without becoming stifling? (See Figure 1.) Each couple must face this crucial question individually. Unfortunately, all too many couples find it difficult to strike this balance. The first step is recognition that this situation can be a real problem. This step alone demands maximum insight on the part of both patient and partner. The patient must deal with denial, avoidance, fear, and rebellion; the partner must temper good intentions and avoid becoming overbearing and rigid. Sometimes it's better for a spouse to ease up and accept some deviations from a plan in order for the patient to sustain independence and self-esteem, even if the actions appear immature and potentially harmful. Yet a spouse should not turn a blind eye to avoidance and deviation from a medical plan. Often a doctor and/or counselor can help a couple successfully navigate this new aspect of their partnership.

In Stanley's case, his doctor advised couples counseling as part of the overall treatment program. This helped, but Stanley and Marilyn had a good deal of work to do to repair their relationship. Stanley needed to assume more responsibility for his health, and Marilyn had to recognize that there were some aspects of her husband's lifestyle that she could not control. "We still don't have all the answers," she confesses, "but we're now able to talk about our fears and other feelings."

TAKING CONTROL

There are many ways to modify the harmful effects of stress. Regular exercise, especially at the beginning of the day, is an excellent way of countering stress and at the same time improving heart health. In certain instances medication may be required to counter stress and anxiety. (This should be discussed with your doctor.) Group therapy, a common component of many cardiac rehab programs; psychotherapy or psychological counseling; and behavior modification can all help keep stress from becoming overwhelming. Building (or rebuilding) a network of supportive relationships is critical. Some people who live alone or lack human companionship often turn to a pet as a buffer against stress. In fact, a number of studies confirm that having a companion animal can help lower blood pressure and modify other risk factors, including stress. You might consider adopting a pet if the circumstances seem right for you.

Various behavior modification techniques are known to help counter stress. One of the easiest and most studied is the relaxation response, a set of exercises

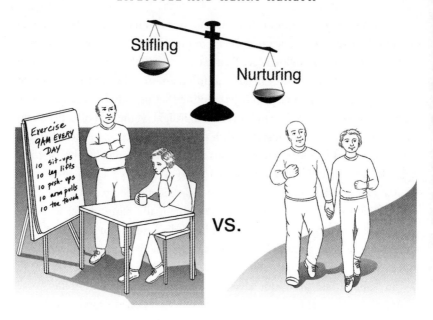

FIGURE 1. A better way. It's often hard to avoid becoming rigid and domineering when a loved one has trouble making needed lifestyle changes. But through communication and positive involvement, it's possible to both help your partner and preserve the family peace.

devised by Dr. Herbert Benson of Harvard University (see Box 8). It has been shown to counteract the effects of the "fight-or-flight" response to stress.

Other relaxation techniques include yoga, tai chi, transcendental meditation, aromatherapy, music, massage, and many others. Some of these are ancient techniques that originated as components of traditional Asian culture and medicine. In recent years, they have become increasingly common in the United States and other Western societies. They can be learned in classes, which are now widely available, or with books or videos. Other popular behavior modification techniques include biofeedback training, anxiety management training, and anger management training. These techniques usually are taught by psychologists or other mental health professionals who have undergone special training. Some cardiac rehab programs now offer them; they are also taught at mental health clinics, medical centers, and various other settings. Ask your doctor or a mental health professional for recommendations, and before undergoing training, check the practitioner's credentials.

Box 8

THE RELAXATION RESPONSE

There are several variations of the "relaxation response" technique, but all involve progressive muscle relaxation and deep breathing.

1. Sit quietly in a comfortable chair, with feet resting on the floor and arms relaxed in your lap or on the armrest. There should be no undue muscular strain on any part of the body. Turn off any lights, radio, TV, or other distractions.

2. Close your eyes.

3. Tense and then relax your foot muscles, and, then progressing upward, tense and then relax the muscles in your legs, torso, arms, neck, and finally your face and scalp. Keep the muscles loose and relaxed after tensing.

4. While relaxing your muscles, continue to breathe through your nose. Strive for natural, even breaths, and as you become aware of your breathing, say a short phrase or single world silently to yourself each time you exhale. The repetition of the word or phrase helps break the train of distracting thoughts.

5. Continue in this relaxed position, with eyes closed, muscles loose, and breathing evenly, for ten minutes (or longer if desired).

6. Throughout, strive to adopt a passive attitude. If distracting thoughts intervene, disregard them and redirect your attention to the repetition of the word or phrase.

7. At the end of the time, sit quietly for a few more minutes, at first with your eyes closed and then with them open.

Biofeedback Training

Through biofeedback training, individuals learn to control certain stress-related physical responses. In the training sessions, which are offered at many mental health clinics and clinical psychology programs at most medical centers, sensors are attached to various parts of the body to measure the body's response to stressful challenges. For example, subjects may be shown a picture or subjected to a sound that typically raises blood pressure and speeds the heart rate. By watching signals on a monitor, the subject tries to control these responses. After learning how to manipulate these normally involuntary body responses, the person can then use the technique to manage stressful situations encountered in daily life.

Anxiety Management Training

The training for anxiety management is a three-stage program designed to teach stress management skills that can be used in almost any tension-producing situation. Participants are taught to modulate responses to stress by practicing guided imagery—concentration on a word, color, or visual scene that invokes a feeling of calm—as well as relaxation techniques to modulate responses to stress. For example, a person who constantly feels under time pressure, often consulting a clock and then fretting over the passing minutes, may be taught to associate a clock instead with a calming image, such as waves gently breaking on the beach. The imagery, combined with deep breathing or other relaxation techniques, has been shown to control the sudden rises in blood pressure that often accompany stress.

Anger Management Training

Also referred to as *stress inoculation therapy,* anger management training is designed to modify feelings of anger and hostility. It involves teaching coping skills in three phases: learning to focus on responses to anger-arousing situations and discriminating between a positive and detrimental display of anger; using coping strategies such as meditation or relaxation exercises to replace angry thoughts; and finally, expressing negative sentiments without antagonizing others. Training typically involves role-playing, in which a therapist teaches the participant how to manage anger and negative responses to it.

THE ROLE OF DEPRESSION

In any given year, about 5 to 10 percent of American adults suffer from a bout of clinical depression; among those who have a heart attack, the percentage zooms to one-third. Unfortunately, most of these patients go undiagnosed and untreated or undertreated, possibly increasing their cardiovascular risk. Interviews with patients who have suffered a heart attack or undergone treatments such as coronary bypass surgery often reveal that depression either predated the problem or developed shortly thereafter. Gerald, a sixty-three-year-old mechanical engineer, is typical of such patients. He suffered a mild heart attack and before leaving the hospital underwent triple bypass surgery. Although he seemingly made a good recovery from both the heart attack and surgery, he had difficulty picking up the threads of his previous life. He spent most of his time staring into space or sleeping. His cardiologist found no physical explanation for Gerald's lethargy, and his wife finally convinced him to seek referral to a mental health professional. Tests indicated that Gerald's depression did not begin with his heart attack; instead, many of the symptoms he now suffered were probably present well before that. He had lost interest in his job and most of the activities he had once enjoyed; in fact, his once optimistic outlook had turned to one of persistent pessimism. He also recalled difficulty sleeping and an unexplained weight gain.

What, if any, role this depression played in Gerald's heart attack is unknown; but there is little doubt that depression and anxiety disorders influence heart disease and its outcome. A number of studies conducted in the last few decades have shown that depression greatly worsens the outlook of heart patients and may also increase or exacerbate other risk factors. One of these studies, published by the Centers for Disease Control and Prevention, followed three thousand men for sixteen years. Initially, all the participants had normal blood pressure, but those who suffered from episodes of clinical depression or severe anxiety were two to three times more likely to develop high blood pressure than their counterparts who did not experience these psychological disorders.

The Johns Hopkins Precursors Study followed almost 1,200 medical students for forty years. During that time, 12 percent had at least one episode of clinical depression, and these subjects had a significantly higher incidence of coronary artery disease than did their counterparts who did not become depressed. A study conducted by a New York labor union program assessed five thousand participants with high blood pressure and also screened them for depression. The study found that those diagnosed with depression had twice the risk of a heart attack compared to participants who were hypertensive but not depressed.

Although depression appears to increase risk in both men and women, some studies suggest that the effect is greater in men. A long-term study by the National Health and Nutrition Examination Survey (NHANES I) found that women had a higher incidence of depression than men. The cardiovascular death rate among males, however, was higher than that of females. Still, the influence on women was significant: those women who suffered from depression had twice the incidence of heart disease compared to those women who were not depressed.

How Depression Affects the Heart

Although much remains to be learned about the links between depression and heart disease, a number of studies conducted in the last decade point to multiple effects on the cardiovascular system. One of these, changes in heart rhythm, was documented by Duke University Medical Center. Researchers there screened seventy-two heart attack patients for depression and anxiety and found that 18 percent were clinically depressed. Of these, almost 40 percent suffered at least one episode of a serious cardiac arrhythmia (ventricular tachycardia), compared to 10 percent of the other patients. Because this type of arrhythmia increases the risk of death after a heart attack, the study concluded that screening for and treating depression can significantly improve the outlook of heart attack patients.

A number of studies have also linked depression and anxiety disorders with an increased risk of high blood pressure—an independent cardiovascular risk factor. Exactly if (or how) depression may raise blood pressure is unknown, although studies have found that depression and anxiety can elevate levels of stress hormones (for example, adrenaline and cortisol) that, in turn, increase blood pressure. Recent studies have also implicated depression in elevated insulin and cholesterol levels (perhaps because of hormonal changes that accompany depression), as well as in changes in blood clotting.

Sources of Depression

Many people mistakenly regard depression as something to be endured—they resist seeking help because they feel they can get over it on their own. But trying to "tough it out" can be a fatal mistake, especially among persons who have already been diagnosed with heart disease or those who are at high risk of developing it. Although depression strikes people of all ages and backgrounds, it is more common among people who have suffered a heart attack, stroke, or other major illness. It also commonly develops following coronary bypass surgery and other treatments. Certain medications, such as beta blockers, can also trigger or worsen depression.

Are you at risk for depression? It is essential to recognize the warning signs (see Box 9). If you do seek treatment, the most effective therapy for depression entails both medication and professional counseling. One class of antidepressant drugs known as selective serotonin reuptake inhibitors (SSRIs) can be helpful—SSRIs include such medications as fluoxetine (Prozac) or paroxetine (Paxil). These drugs also affect platelet function, helping to keep blood from clotting.

Depression often cannot be dealt with adequately by either a primary care physician or cardiologist; treatment by a psychiatrist or psychologist may be required. But simply recognizing the problem and doing something—indeed, almost anything—will help. Regular exercise, for example, can help overcome mild depression, presumably by stimulating the brain to release endorphins, the

---

Box 9

SYMPTOMS OF DEPRESSION

A diagnosis of depression should be suspected if five or more of the following symptoms are present daily for two weeks and interfere with routine daily activities.

- Persistent sad, anxious, or empty mood
- Feelings of restlessness and irritability
- Feelings of hopelessness and/or pessimism
- Feelings of guilt, worthlessness, or helplessness
- Loss of interest or pleasure in activities that were once enjoyed, including sex
- Decreased energy, persistent fatigue, or feelings of being slowed down
- Difficulty concentrating, remembering, or making decisions
- Changes in sleep patterns, such as insomnia or excessive sleeping
- Changes in appetite and/or weight
- Thoughts of death or suicide; attempted suicide

---

body's natural mood enhancers. Many people advocate herbal remedies, such as St. John's wort. (A word of warning, however: Check with your doctor before taking any herbal or nutritional supplement because many of these may interact with your other medications.) Many studies show that simply taking a placebo (a sugar pill) can produce positive results if the person adheres to the "regimen" and thinks he or she is getting the real thing. This is but another example of the little-understood ways in which the brain plays an instrumental role in the healing process.

ROLE OF ANXIETY

The possible role of anxiety disorders in cardiovascular disease is less clear-cut than that of stress or depression. For example, many people who suffer from panic attacks are convinced that they have heart disease because the symptoms of a panic attack—chest pain, shortness of breath, a sense of impending doom, among others—are hard to distinguish from those of a heart attack. Every day, dozens of Americans are rushed to emergency rooms because of suspected heart attacks

Box 10

PHOBIC DISORDER SELF-TEST

The Nurses' Health Study used the following questions to assess the level of phobic anxiety. Answers were ranked as never/not at all, sometimes/moderately, or often/very/yes. The level of anxiety was classified into four groups, ranging from zero to four; those with the highest scores had the greatest number of cardiac deaths or events.

- Do you have an unreasonable fear of being in enclosed spaces such as shops, elevators, etc.?
- Do you find yourself worrying about getting some incurable illness?
- Are you afraid of heights?
- Do you feel panicky in crowds?
- Do you worry unduly when relatives are late coming home?
- Do you feel more relaxed indoors?
- Do you dislike going out alone?
- Do you feel uneasy traveling on buses or trains, even if they are not crowded?

only to find out that their symptoms are instead due to anxiety or a panic attack. Obviously, it's always better to err on the side of safety, but a person with a history of panic attacks may be well advised to seek treatment of this anxiety disorder rather than dwell on the possibility that something is wrong with the heart.

There seem to be exceptions to this generalization. Studies indicate that women who suffer from phobic anxiety do, indeed, have an increased risk of sudden cardiac death and heart attacks. In one of the most extensive studies, the Nurses' Health Study at Boston's Brigham and Women's Hospital and Massachusetts General Hospital, more than 72,000 nurses, aged thirty to fifty-five years, have been followed for twelve years. In a 2005 report, the researchers found that phobic anxiety is as dangerous a cardiovascular risk factor as is smoking, body weight, or a sedentary lifestyle. Specifically, over the twelve-year follow-up, study participants who suffered from phobic disorders suffered 97 sudden cardiac deaths, 267 deaths from coronary heart disease, and 930 nonfatal heart attacks. Overall, women with high levels of phobic anxiety were four times more likely to die suddenly of heart disease than were women who ranked on the lowest quarter of the anxiety scale.

These findings are especially important for women because they are more vulnerable to anxiety disorders than men. It is estimated that 5 percent of American adults suffer from some form of anxiety disorder, and as many as 15 percent of these have phobic anxiety (see Box 10 for a phobic disorder self-test). Dr. Christine M. Albert, assistant professor at Harvard Medical School and lead author of this Nurses' Health Study report, noted: "Researchers and clinicians still do not know all the risk factors and potential triggers of sudden cardiac death. These results . . . point to one possible risk factor and should prompt physicians to be aware of this risk when treating patients with phobic disorders."

SUMMING UP

We are only beginning to understand the importance of the mind-body connection for overall health and heart disease in particular. But given what we do know, it's safe to say that the mind plays a more critical role in maintaining heart health than had been assumed even a decade ago. So if stress, depression, and certain types of anxiety raise cardiovascular risk, it may well be that more positive psychological factors—for example, hope and optimism—are protective. This is why we contend that knowledge and a positive, can-do attitude are important aspects of your lifelong health-care program.

5

Controlling and Stopping Smoking

Cigarette smoking is by far the leading cause of preventable mortality in the United States, accounting for about 440,000 premature deaths a year. By now, everyone is well aware of the role smoking plays in the development of lung cancer and other pulmonary diseases. But despite all the publicity of recent years, many Americans either do not know or ignore the fact that cigarettes also damage the cardiovascular system and are a major risk factor for heart attacks.

Numerous studies confirm that smoking greatly accelerates coronary artery disease and the buildup of fatty deposits in blood vessels (atherosclerosis). The precise mechanisms have yet to be defined, but researchers have identified a number of possibilities. For example, smoking increases levels of carbon monoxide in the blood, which can damage the artery lining and contribute to atherosclerosis. Smoking also appears to lower HDL, the good cholesterol, and increase LDL, the harmful cholesterol. In addition, smoking raises blood levels of fibrinogen, a substance instrumental in blood clotting, which can lead to a heart attack or stroke. Nicotine raises blood pressure and heart rate, while constricting the coronary arteries. This effect not only increases the heart's workload, but it also reduces the amount of oxygen reaching the heart muscle, which can lead to angina, or chest pain, caused by ischemia (insufficient blood supply to the heart muscle). Finally, nicotine can provoke disturbances in the heart's normal rhythm.

Some people mistakenly think they can reduce their cardiovascular risk by switching to a low-tar, low-nicotine cigarette or smoking a pipe or cigars instead of cigarettes. Not so; when it comes to heart health, there is no such thing as safe tobacco. There is good news, however: smokers who quit can halt or even reverse many of these adverse effects. Even people who smoke two packs a day can see their cardiovascular mortality risk begin to drop in a year or so and will reach the level of nonsmokers in five to ten years after stopping. (The same is not true for lung cancer and many other smoking-related diseases.) But you don't have to wait this long to reap real benefits from stopping smoking. Just twenty minutes after smoking your last cigarette, the nicotine-induced constriction of the peripheral blood vessels eases, allowing blood pressure to drop. In about eight hours, blood oxygen levels return to normal, and carbon monoxide levels begin to drop. Smell and taste begin to return to normal, so you can once again enjoy the flavor of food. Metabolism also returns to normal. These changes may account for the modest weight gain that many people experience when they stop smoking. Indeed, many smokers, especially young women, resist quitting because they fear gaining weight. Although it's true that many people do gain a few pounds when they stop smoking, this is not a valid reason to continue—or start—smoking. Tobacco use is much more harmful than being overweight. The weight gain can be minimized by paying attention to diet and increasing exercise, which also helps reduce the nervousness that some people experience when they attempt to stop. In fact, if you are both overweight and smoke, don't try to correct both problems at the same time. Stop smoking first and then tackle the weight problem.

Smoking affects virtually every part of the body. It causes premature skin wrinkling, especially in women, and men may develop erectile dysfunction. Smoking accelerates the bone loss of osteoporosis, and women who smoke typically enter menopause several years earlier than nonsmokers; it can also cause fertility problems in both men and women. (Other reasons to stop smoking are summarized in Box 11.)

OVERCOMING NICOTINE ADDICTION

As anyone who has ever tried to stop smoking will readily testify, it's not easy. This is because nicotine is as addictive as heroin and cocaine, according to some studies. Consequently, stopping results in unpleasant withdrawal symptoms, which appear to be more intense in women than men. But these symptoms gradually lessen and usually disappear in a week or two.

Box 11

REASONS TO QUIT SMOKING

These are just some of the many good rationales for stopping smoking. We're sure you can think of others.

1. Add years to your life
2. Help avoid heart attacks, lung cancer, emphysema, and bronchitis
3. Give your heart and circulatory system a break
4. Get rid of smokers' cough
5. Improve your stamina and feel more vigorous while exercising and participating in sports
6. Stop smoke-related headaches and stomach problems
7. Regain your sense of smell and taste
8. End cigarette breath and get rid of smoke odor on clothes, in your car, and in your home
9. Save money
10. Avoid exposing family members and others to your secondhand smoke, which is harmful to their health
11. Get rid of stains on your teeth and fingers
12. Get rid of messy ashtrays, ashes on carpets, and burns in clothing and furniture
13. Set a good example for others, especially your children
14. Prove your self-control and willpower

Source: Adapted from "7-Day Plan to Help You Stop Smoking Cigarettes," American Cancer Society.

As might be expected, people who start smoking at an early age and then continue cigarette use for a number of years have the hardest time stopping. This was certainly the case for Sam, our fifty-two-year-old school bus driver. He got hooked on cigarettes at the age of thirteen—the age when the greatest number of youngsters start smoking—and by the time he finished high school, he was going through two packs a day. Over the years he made a number of half-hearted attempts to stop, but within a week or two, he'd be back to his two packs a day. He seldom exercised and was moderately overweight.

When Sam started experiencing chest pains while walking up a flight of stairs, his wife feared that he was a candidate for a heart attack, an especially worrisome prospect because his job entailed driving dozens of children to and from school each day. She insisted that he see a doctor, who determined that Sam had high blood cholesterol, type II diabetes, and high blood pressure—all serious risk factors for heart disease exacerbated by his smoking and sedentary lifestyle. Medication soon brought his blood cholesterol, diabetes, and high blood pressure under control, but his doctor warned that these measures were not enough; it was also imperative that he stop smoking. After questioning Sam about his reasons for smoking and past history of unsuccessful attempts to stop, the doctor suggested that he try stopping "cold turkey" and use a nicotine patch or gum to ease him through the withdrawal period. Sam selected nicotine gum, which seemed to work for a few weeks. But when Sam tried to cut back on the gum, he encountered a major stumbling block. He simply could not wean himself off the gum; in fact, he realized that he was popping in a new stick before the old one was chewed out. His doctor had warned him that overuse of nicotine was itself a danger, so he tried switching to a nicotine patch regimen that gradually lowered the dosage over a period of time. It required tremendous willpower to stop the gum, which gave him a quick "fix," but his doctor had warned him of the danger of a nicotine overdose when chewing nicotine gum while wearing a patch. So instead of nicotine gum he switched to a sugar-free spicy gum that seemed to satisfy his need to chew something as a substitute for the cigarettes. The entire process took almost six months, but Sam was finally able to stop the patches. "I still want a cigarette every now and then, especially after dinner or when I'm in a room where someone else is smoking," Sam told his doctor. "But I'm determined not to backslide."

After Sam was finally off cigarettes, the doctor encouraged him to tackle his weight problem. (Again, although being overweight also raises cardiovascular risk, if you are both overweight and smoke, don't try to correct both problems at the same time. Stop smoking first and then tackle the weight problem.) Sam's wife was a great help with her husband's weight problem. She accompanied Sam to a counseling session with a dietitian, and took over preparing meals that included more vegetables, whole grain products, and lean meats and fish, and less fatty meats, processed foods, and sugar. At her urging, Sam went with her to an animal shelter to look over dogs in need of a home. They ended up adopting Barney, a lively Labrador mix who would need at least two long walks a day. Exercising Barney soon became part of the couple's daily routine—Sam returns home in the mid-morning after dropping off his last busload of schoolchildren, and he then takes Barney for a long walk. After dinner, he and his wife again walk Barney, an activity that has become a favorite part of their day.

At his last checkup, Sam was pleased to learn that his blood pressure, blood sugar, and cholesterol levels were all normal, and that he had shed almost twenty pounds, with another ten to go before achieving his weight goal. "I must confess, I've never felt better," he said recently. "I feel I've been given a new lease on life, and I can now go up two or three flights of stairs and not feel even a tiny twinge."

Nicotine Patches and Gum

To get through the nicotine withdrawal period, many people do what Sam did: turn to other forms of nicotine, such as skin patches or nicotine gum, which are now available over the counter. The skin patches (for example, Habitrol and Nicoderm CQ) allow small amounts of nicotine to be absorbed into tiny blood vessels in the skin; the gum (Nicorette) also provides nicotine that is absorbed through membranes in the mouth. These aids have the advantage of lessening withdrawal symptoms while the smoker adjusts to giving up the other aspects of cigarette use. The body can start recovering from the constant exposure to tar and the many other toxic components of cigarettes without experiencing the unpleasant nicotine withdrawal symptoms encountered in abrupt cessation of smoking.

Typically, the nicotine dosage is gradually reduced over time; for example, full-strength patches may be worn for the first two or three weeks, and then are replaced by patches that deliver lesser amounts. Eventually the goal is to forgo the patches entirely. Ideally, nicotine gum should be approached in the same manner, with a gradual reduction in the amount chewed until the ex-smoker can get by without it entirely. Some people do this by substituting regular chewing gum for every other stick of nicotine gum; others stretch out the time between chews. In any event, it's important to remember that nicotine itself is highly toxic—in fact, it's a common ingredient in rat poison—and caution is needed to avoid an overdose. Never use nicotine patches and gum simultaneously, and abstain from smoking when using either product. Always follow the package directions when using either product, and make a concerted effort to stop them as soon as possible. This may entail switching to a medication or to an alternative therapy such as acupuncture, self-hypnosis, or herbal products.

Other Forms of Nicotine

Some smokers switch from cigarettes to snuff or chewing tobacco in the mistaken belief that these are safer forms of tobacco. Although smokeless tobacco does not expose the body to tar and some of the other harmful components of cigarettes, it is by no means a safe alternative. It contains nicotine and many of the other toxic substances found in cigarettes, and numerous studies link smokeless tobacco to an increased risk of mouth and throat cancer, inflamed gums (gingivitis), as well as severe gum disease and tooth loss.

Helpful Medications

In addition to nicotine products, prescription medications can be helpful in countering withdrawal symptoms while quitting. Of these, Zyban (buproprion) is one of the most widely prescribed. Zyban is actually a repackaged form of Wellbutrin, an antidepressant that has largely been replaced by newer drugs that inhibit the brain's uptake of serotonin (for example, Zoloft or Prozac). Patients taking Wellbutrin to treat depression often reported a lessened desire to smoke. Clinical studies confirmed that the drug relieved nicotine withdrawal symptoms, so Wellbutrin was reformulated into Zyban and marketed as a smoking-cessation aid.

Smokers are instructed to start taking Zyban while they are still smoking, but to pick a firm date to quit within two or three weeks. By the time the date arrives, many smokers are already experiencing a lessened desire to smoke. After they stop, the drug appears to be most effective in reducing feelings of irritability, frustration, anger, anxiety, depression, and restlessness—all common nicotine withdrawal symptoms.

As with any medication, Zyban can cause unwanted side effects. The most common are dry mouth and difficulty sleeping; it can also cause tremors, confusion, and a rash. Anyone experiencing these effects should contact a doctor as soon as possible; the drug may need to be stopped or the dosage changed. In addition, Zyban should not be used by persons who have a seizure disorder (epilepsy) or eating disorder (bulimia or anorexia nervosa) because of an increased risk of seizures; it also should not be used by persons taking a monoamine oxidase (MAO) inhibitor or those undergoing withdrawal from other addictions, especially to alcohol or benzodiazepines—for example, diazepam (Valium)—and other sedatives.

Other antidepressants, especially serotonin reuptake inhibitors, may also lessen symptoms of nicotine withdrawal. Herbal products that have effects similar to SSRIs, such as St. John's wort, may also be helpful, but this benefit has not been proven in clinical studies. There are also herbal products designed specifically to aid in smoking cessation; these include Nicocure and Final Smoke, both mixtures of a number of herbs. Check the labels carefully, however, as some con-

Box 12

SELF-ASSESSMENT QUIZ: WHY DO YOU SMOKE?

Here are some statements by people describing why they smoke. How often do you feel this way when smoking? Score yourself by choosing one number for each statement below.

5 = Always 4 = Frequently 3 = Occasionally 2 = Seldom 1 = Never

A. I smoke cigarettes in order to keep myself from slowing down.

B. Handling a cigarette is part of the enjoyment of smoking.

C. Smoking cigarettes is pleasant and relaxing.

D. I light up a cigarette when I feel angry about something.

E. When I am out of cigarettes, I find it almost unbearable until I can get more.

F. I smoke cigarettes automatically without being aware of it.

G. I smoke cigarettes to perk myself up.

H. Part of the enjoyment of smoking comes from the steps I take to light up.

I. I find cigarettes pleasurable.

J. I light up a cigarette when I feel uncomfortable or upset.

K. I am very aware of when I'm not smoking.

L. I light up a cigarette without realizing I still have one burning.

M. I smoke cigarettes to give myself a "lift."

N. When I smoke, part of the enjoyment is watching the smoke as I exhale it.

O. I want a cigarette most when I'm comfortable and relaxed.

P. When I feel "blue" or want to take my mind off something, I smoke a cigarette.

Q. I feel a real gnawing need or yearning for a cigarette when I haven't smoked for a while.

R. I've found a cigarette in my mouth and didn't remember putting it there.

How to Score

1. Enter the numbers you chose in the appropriate spaces below (putting the number you selected for question A on line A, for question B on line B, and so on).

2. Add the three scores on each line to get your total score for each category. For example, the sum of the scores for lines A, G, and M gives you your score on Stimulation. Scores of 11 or more indicate that this factor is an important source of satisfaction; scores of between 7 and 11 indicate less importance; and scores of 7 or less are low and probably show that this factor does not apply to you.

(A)_____ + (G)_____ + (M)_____ = _____ (Stimulation)

(B)_____ + (H)_____ + (N)_____ = _____(Handling)

(C)_____ + (I)_____ + (O)_____ = _____(Relaxation)

(D)_____ + (J)_____ + (P)_____ = _____(Crutch)

(E)_____ + (K)_____ + (Q)_____ = _____(Craving)

(F)_____ + (L)_____ + (R)_____ = _____(Habit)

What a High Score Means and What You Can Do

Stimulation. You smoke because it gives you a lift. Substitute a brisk walk or a few simple exercises.

Handling. You like the ritual and trappings of smoking. Find other ways to keep your hands busy.

Relaxation. You get a real sense of pleasure from smoking. An honest consideration of the harmful effects may dampen the pleasure.

Crutch. If you light up most often up when you're angry or depressed, you're using smoking as a tranquilizer. In a tough situation, take a deep breath to relax, call a friend, and talk over your feelings. If you can learn new ways to cope, you're on your way to quitting.

Craving. Quitting smoking is difficult for you if you are dependent on nicotine, but once you've stopped, it will be possible to resist the temptation to smoke because the withdrawal effort is too tough to face again.

Habit. If you usually smoke without even realizing you're doing it, you should find it easy to break the habit pattern. Start by asking: "Do I really want this cigarette?" Change smoking patterns and make cigarettes hard to get at.

Adapted from "7-Day Plan to Help You Stop Smoking Cigarettes," American Cancer Society, and Daniel Horn, Ph.D., Director of the National Clearinghouse for Smoking and Health, Public Health Service, "Smoker's Self-Test."

tain licorice root and other herbs that can raise blood pressure or cause other problems. It's a good idea to talk to your health-care provider or pharmacist before trying an herbal remedy, especially if you are taking other medications.

HOW TO STOP SMOKING

An individualized approach is needed for the difficult task of quitting smoking, just as it is for all the other changes suggested in this book. There is no single smoking cessation method that works for everyone, and finding the one that will most likely bring success starts with a thoughtful assessment of your current lifestyle and personality. (For a good self-assessment quiz, see Box 12.)

For most people, quitting "cold turkey," rather than tapering off, seems to work best. For others, however, a gradual reduction—perhaps dropping two or three cigarettes a day—brings success and may reduce withdrawal symptoms. In any event, the goal must be to stop completely.

Although many people manage to quit on their own, others need a structured program or aids, such as hypnosis, acupuncture, or perhaps medication. There are commercial programs, such as SmokEnders, and a number of organizations, including the American Heart Association and American Cancer Society, conduct periodic smoking cessation clinics and workshops. Some workplaces, as well as many local hospitals, also offer stop-smoking programs and clinics. In fact, some health plans cover the costs of smoking cessation programs, so check your policy or contact your health-care administrator for guidance.

Regardless of the method you select, a strong support system will help you succeed. For example, it's difficult to quit if your colleagues, spouse, or others with whom you maintain close contact continue to smoke. (See Box 13 for more tips for quitting.) Try recruiting the smokers in your life to join your efforts and lend their support; at the very least, ask them to refrain from smoking in your presence. As an added incentive, make copies of the box "Reasons to Quit Smoking," then post them on your refrigerator, mirror, and other prominent places where you will see the list whenever you feel the urge for a cigarette.

SUMMING UP

If you smoke, there's no doubt that stopping will benefit your overall health and help reduce your risk of a heart attack and other serious diseases. But most smokers find that stopping is difficult at best and many insist they simply can't wean themselves off nicotine—a powerful addictive substance. Smoking cessation is

Box 13

TIPS FOR QUITTING

1. Make a list of reasons to quit and the benefits you'll get from doing so. Read the list at least once a day, and add to it as you go along.

2. Use the accompanying Smoking Self-Assessment Quiz to analyze why you smoke. This can help you identify the method that is likely to work best for you.

3. Pick a date for stopping. It might be the American Cancer Society's Great American Smokeout, your birthday, or any other day that's important to you. But strive to find a time when you're not under a lot of stress from other sources.

4. Enlist the help of those close to you. Ask those who smoke not to do so in your presence.

5. Get ready to stop by switching to a brand that's not as appealing as your regular choice. Buy only one pack, and when that one is gone, switch to another, even less appealing brand. Stop carrying matches or a lighter, and keep cigarettes in a place that's not readily accessible. Start getting rid of ashtrays and start limiting the places where you can smoke. For example, put your home, car, and workplace off-limits to smoking. (In many states and localities, it's already illegal to smoke in most public indoor places.)

6. Get two large jars. In one, collect all your butts. In the other, collect money equal to that which you're spending on cigarettes. As you quit, continue to add the money you normally would have spent. When you finally stop, you can use the money to reward yourself with a special treat.

7. The first few days of abstaining from smoking are the hardest, so make every effort to avoid the situations in which you would normally smoke. For example, if you usually have a cigarette after a meal, take a walk instead.

8. Keep your hands and mouth busy, especially during the first difficult days. Stock up on low-calorie snacks, such as carrot and celery sticks or fruits; chew gum (including nicotine gum if you're really having difficulty quitting); or suck on a toothpick or a straw.

9. Instead of focusing on your desire for a cigarette, concentrate on enjoying the benefits of not smoking. Increase your exercise and marvel at how you have more energy and are not so short of breath. Brush your teeth or

(continued)

(Box 8 *continued*)

rinse with mouthwash several times a day to savor a fresh-tasting mouth. Savor your renewed taste of food and now and then indulge in a special treat, such as a piece of (heart-healthy) dark chocolate.

Source: Adapted from B. L. Zaret, M. Moser, and L. S. Cohen, eds., *Yale University School of Medicine Heart Book* (New York: Hearst Books, 1992).

one area in which the adage "If at first you don't succeed, try, try again" certainly applies. Few people manage to stop on their first attempt. But as any ex-smoker will tell you, your chances of success increase with each try, so don't be discouraged if you initially fall back into your old smoking habit. Just start again, knowing that with fresh determination and a strong support system, your chances of success are increased—and that your success will yield major health dividends.

II

The
Basics
of
Lifelong
Treatment

Lifelong heart care involves not only the lifestyle changes described in the previous chapters, but also proper diagnosis and, when appropriate, medical treatment for your specific cardiovascular disease. Obviously, any diagnostic or treatment program must take into consideration your individual circumstances and be prescribed and overseen by a physician. As stressed in previous chapters, early diagnosis and treatment often can slow or even prevent the progression of disease. So if you are found to have what was once considered mild high blood pressure or borderline elevated blood cholesterol or blood sugar levels, treatment at this stage may forestall the need for later more invasive or aggressive treatments.

Success depends on setting realistic goals and then following through on working to achieve these goals. This is why it is so important that you establish a close working relationship with your doctor and that you have a supportive environment in which you can best maintain appropriate lifestyle modifications and follow your individualized lifelong heart-care program.

As we stress repeatedly, there are no quick fixes; instead, achieving and maintaining heart health is a lifelong endeavor. Of course, there are some conditions that can be remedied by surgery or other interventions. But as with drug therapy, these are unlikely to cure the underlying problem. While we cannot hold out the promise of a cure, a lifelong, sustainable program can produce renewed energy and zest for life as well as additional years of productive and enjoyable living. So from our perspective, we can emphatically say that adopting the lifestyle changes is well worth the effort. But this may only be one step.

In Part II, we provide a broad overview of the various tests and medical treatments used for the more common heart conditions. Here we give you explanations in "broad strokes": our categories of diagnostic studies and treatments are not designed to provide detailed or comprehensive guidelines for how to approach your medical care. Do not use the information to alter your doctor's prescribed regimen; instead, use it as a basis for discussions with your doctor. Many patients hesitate to ask questions or raise concerns with their doctors, fearing that somehow their questions will be resented. On the contrary, most doctors welcome engaging in a dialogue with patients, and recognize that a well-informed and engaged patient is likely to follow a long-term regimen and enjoy an improved outcome.

CHAPTER

6

Diagnostic Tests and Procedures

The many advances in medical technology of recent decades have revolutionized the diagnosis of cardiovascular disease. Not long ago, a cardiovascular workup was pretty much limited to a physical exam, listening to heart and lung sounds through a stethoscope, and a few basic tests including an electrocardiogram (ECG or EKG), blood pressure measurement, and perhaps a chest X-ray. Today we have an array of sophisticated tests that allow us to view the heart in action and assess how it is functioning; look into the heart, coronary arteries, and other blood vessels; and quickly home in on the nature of myriad problems with amazing accuracy. Technology and treatments are changing quickly, with new tests and advances in treatments being introduced at an increasingly rapid rate.

The precise sequence of tests is dictated by your initial symptoms and history as well as risk factors, age, overall health, occupation, individual preferences, and other idiosyncrasies. The immediate circumstances are also important. For example, a person experiencing a heart attack may be rushed to a special laboratory for immediate interventional procedures that include cardiac catheterization—the threading of a narrow catheter into the heart's coronary arteries—followed by urgent treatment, such as coronary angiography or bypass surgery. In contrast, cardiac catheterization may be a later test in a person with mild symptoms or risk factors. (Box 14 describes a typical case history, offering a possible sequence of symptoms, diagnostic tests, and treatment.)

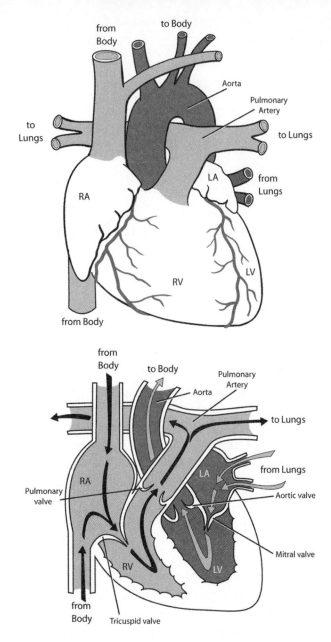

FIGURE 2. Anatomy of the heart. The drawing on the top illustrates the major vessels that carry blood to and from the heart, as well as the coronary arteries, which nourish the heart muscle. The drawing on the bottom shows the path of oxygen-depleted blood flowing to the right atrium (RA), then to the right ventricle (RV) and into the lungs. After picking up a fresh supply of oxygen, the blood returns to the left atrium (LA), passes into the left ventricle (LV), and is then pumped into the aorta to enter the body's circulatory system.

THE MEDICAL HISTORY

The medical history is one of the most important components of a medical checkup. If you are seeing a doctor for the first time, it is especially important that you describe any past or current illnesses. Be prepared to describe the medical histories of close relatives. Do you have a family history of heart disease? Diabetes? High blood pressure? Stroke? Cancer? Allergies? Rare or heredity diseases? You should also be ready to list all your medications, including nonprescription drugs, nutritional supplements, and any natural or alternative medicines. In fact, it's a good idea to take all your medications with you so your doctor can tell exactly what you're taking. You will need to tell the doctor about any troubling symptoms, including sexual problems and other intimate details of your life. Erectile dysfunction (impotence) in men may be an early indication of diabetes or coronary artery disease. Many people withhold such information, thinking that it's unimportant or that if something is amiss, the doctor will detect it. Or perhaps they find it difficult or embarrassing to discuss private matters. But if your doctor is to get a complete picture of your state of health, it's important for you to give as much information as possible.

THE CARDIOVASCULAR PHYSICAL EXAM

Typically, a doctor begins a cardiovascular workup by measuring your height and weight and doing a careful visual check. Is the skin tone normal? Flushed? Pale? Bluish? The doctor then checks your vital signs. Blood pressure is measured while you sit quietly. A high reading may indicate high blood pressure or hypertension, a condition in which the heart is working overly hard to pump blood through small arteries that are constricted and putting up too much resistance. Or it may simply mean you're nervous being in a doctor's office (a common condition referred to as white-coat hypertension) or that you're still experiencing the effects of a cigarette or cup of coffee (or other jolt of caffeine). In fact, you should wait at least thirty minutes to measure your blood pressure after consuming caffeine or smoking a cigarette. At any rate, if the blood pressure reading is high, it should be repeated later in the exam and at a subsequent visit.

Next, the doctor checks different pulses to learn more about your heart rate. Is it strong and steady? Too fast? Slow? Irregular? Pulses will be checked in different parts of the body—the wrist, above the elbow, both sides of the neck, the groin, behind the knees, and both ankles—because a pulse may be normal in one place and weak or abnormal in another. The doctor will pay particular at-

Box 14

A CASE HISTORY DEMONSTRATING A TYPICAL PROGRESSION
OF DIAGNOSTIC STUDIES AND TREATMENT

David, a fifty-two-year-old lawyer, is a recently divorced father of two who considers himself basically healthy. He leads an active life, playing tennis or golf most weekends and working out at his gym at least two or three times a week. He has a history of high blood pressure, which is controlled by medication, and his LDL cholesterol, at 140 mg/dl, is elevated. He is an ex-smoker and at one time he was about twenty pounds over his ideal weight, but he lost the excess pounds a few years ago and has managed to keep them off.

A few weeks ago, he started experiencing a vague feeling of tightness and mild shortness of breath while working out at the gym. At first he tried to ignore the symptoms, attributing them to stress from his work and family problems. But he also knew that his family history put him in a high-risk category—his father had suffered a fatal heart attack at the young age of forty-nine and his mother died of a stroke when she was sixty-one. So he made an appointment to see his doctor.

The doctor started with a careful physical exam that included blood pressure measurement, an ECG, blood tests, and a chest X-ray. She also recommended an exercise nuclear stress test. During the exercise portion, David started to experience chest pain and shortness of breath, which were relieved after the doctor stopped the test and gave him a nitroglycerine pill. There were also suspicious ECG changes, and the nuclear imaging showed that part of his heart muscle was not getting enough blood. Based on this experience, the doctor recommended that David go to the hospital for cardiac catheterization and coronary angiography—special X-rays of the heart's blood vessels. These tests detected a narrowing in one of David's major coronary arteries. He then underwent angioplasty, a treatment to flatten the fatty deposits (plaque) that were clogging the artery, followed by insertion of a stent, a device to keep the artery open. Within a couple of weeks, David was able to resume his normal activities. His doctor prescribed medication to lower his LDL cholesterol, as well as clopidogrel (Plavix), a drug that helps prevent blood clots and clumping of platelets. The doctor also recommended that he also enroll in a cardiac rehabilitation program that included stress management, dietary counseling, and exercise advice. This program stressed the importance of following a lifelong program that included periodic checkups and special attention to preventing progression of his coronary disease.

David's case illustrates a typical progression of diagnostic tests in a higher-risk patient experiencing mild symptoms. In addition, it shows that even when you take care, your disease may progress. The treatment and outcome are also quite typical and, with David's determination to work with his doctor in following a long-term preventive program, he should enjoy many years of active, productive life. If he had had more extensive coronary artery disease, he may have undergone heart bypass surgery followed by cardiac rehabilitation and medications similar to those his doctor had prescribed.

tention to your blood vessels in the neck. A distended jugular vein may indicate a backup of blood caused by heart failure. A weak pulse or swooshing sound (bruit) in your carotid arteries—the blood vessels on each side of the neck—may be a sign of a blockage in these vital vessels that carry blood to the brain.

Using a stethoscope, the doctor checks the heart and lungs, listening for murmurs, rubs, clicks, gallops, swooshing, or other abnormal sounds. He or she may also listen to sounds in the blood vessels of the neck and other key arteries. The doctor will feel or palpate the abdomen, checking for swellings or possible abnormalities of the liver, spleen, and other internal organs. He will check the extremities for signs of swelling or edema. Swollen ankles, for example, may point to venous insufficiency or a possible sign of heart failure. Disfiguring (or clubbing) of the fingertips raises the suspicion of a circulatory or lung disorder.

Finally, the doctor will dim the lights and use a lighted magnifying instrument to peer into your eyes. This is the only place in the body where small arteries can be viewed directly. Tiny ruptures, narrowing or swelling, tangles, or other abnormalities may indicate damage from high blood pressure, atherosclerosis, or diabetes.

BLOOD AND URINE TESTS

Virtually all physical exams include laboratory evaluations of blood and urine samples (see Table 6). Typically, these tests will provide chemical profiles of specific functions or organ systems. Examples include a lipid profile (with blood drawn after a nine- to twelve-hour fast) to measure total cholesterol as well as a breakdown of LDL, the harmful cholesterol, and HDL, the beneficial cholesterol. Triglycerides, a lipid that is elevated in diabetes and may play a role in atherosclerosis, will be measured, and lipoprotein (a), or Lp(a), a protein molecule that may increase the risk of a heart attack, may also be measured. Other blood tests

TABLE 6

BLOOD AND URINE TESTS IMPORTANT IN A CARDIOVASCULAR WORKUP

Test	What it can tell the doctor
Complete blood count (CBC)	Measures different types of red and white blood cells
Platelet count, fibrinogen, prothrombin time	Helps in the evaluation of bleeding and clotting disorders
Fasting lipid profile	Measures total cholesterol and levels of HDL (the bad cholesterol), LDL (the good cholesterol), and triglycerides
Fasting blood glucose	Measures sugar in blood; screens for diabetes
Insulin levels	Elevated levels may indicate metabolic syndrome (insulin resistance) and increased risk of diabetes
Blood-urea nitrogen (BUN)/ creatinine (Cr)	Measures blood urea nitrogen and creatinine, waste products eliminated by kidney (when elevated, it is a possible sign of kidney malfunction)
Creatine kinase (CK)	Early marker of heart attack or muscle damage; useful in detecting a worrisome side effect of cholesterol-lowering medication (statins)
Creatine kinase MB (CKMB)	Detects heart muscle damage usually caused by a heart attack
Uric acid	Measures waste product of protein metabolism; elevated level may indicate gout or kidney disease
High-sensitivity CRP (hs-CRP)	Measures C-reactive protein to detect inflammation, a newly recognized risk factor for atherosclerosis
Homocysteine	Measures an amino acid involved in protein metabolism; high levels are a cardiovascular risk factor
Hemoglobin A1c	Measure of blood sugar control in diabetes
Liver function tests	Abnormality may indicate heart failure, or side effects of statins (cholesterol-lowering drugs)
Urinalysis	Protein in urine may indicate kidney disorder or heart failure; analysis can also detect bacteria from any urinary tract infection and glucose due to diabetes.

provide important information about other risk factors as well as liver, kidney, endocrine, and other organ function. A routine urinalysis can help detect urinary tract infections and bleeding, kidney disorders, diabetes and other metabolic problems, and dehydration.

THE ELECTROCARDIOGRAM

An electrocardiogram (ECG or EKG) takes about five minutes and can be done in a doctor's office, clinic, or hospital bedside. While you lie quietly on your back, electrodes, or leads, are attached to the chest, arms, and legs. A gel may be applied to the lead sites to improve conduction of the heart's electrical impulses. The impulses are recorded on paper, providing a map of the pathway of the impulses as they move through the heart muscle.

What the results show. An ECG can sometimes help detect blockages in the coronary arteries and help diagnose a heart attack, including a previous silent one, as well as detect a thickening of the heart muscle (hypertrophy) and heart rhythm disturbances. (See Figure 3 for examples.)

Advantages. The test is painless, safe, and inexpensive and can be performed by a technician or nurse. The equipment is widely available in every doctor's office and the results are available immediately. The results also can be transmitted over phone lines for evaluation at a diagnostic center.

Disadvantages. It does not always provide an accurate diagnosis, is often both nonsensitive and nonspecific, and does not predict the likelihood of an impending heart attack. Results can be affected by movement or faulty placement of leads, electrolyte imbalances (too much or too little calcium, potassium, magnesium, or sodium in the blood), a thickening of the heart muscle, medications, and low body temperature, to name but a few factors.

HOLTER MONITOR OR AMBULATORY ECG

This test provides continuous ECG monitoring over twenty-four hours or longer. A portable monitor, typically about the size of a pack of cards, is affixed to ECG leads that are attached to the chest. You will be instructed to carry out normal daily activities and to keep a diary showing the time of exercise, meals, periods of stress, symptoms such as a rapid heartbeat, and other events that may affect results. After the specified time, you will return to a doctor's office or clinic to have the leads and monitor removed, and the ECG recording will be scanned by a computer for abnormalities. There are a number of variations on this test. For

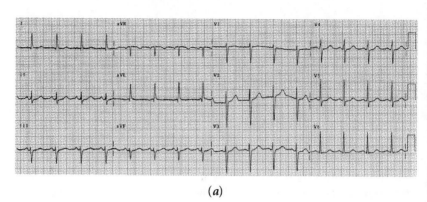

(a)

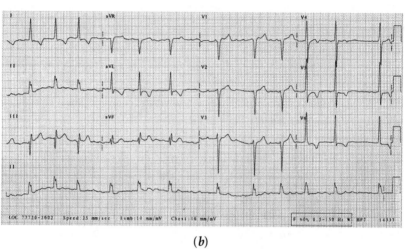

(b)

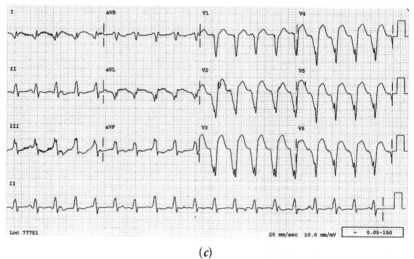

(c)

example, the monitor may be left on for a longer period or periodically activated only during symptoms to record episodes of irregularities. Results can also be transmitted via telephone. An implantable loop recorder may be placed surgically under the skin for extensive periods and can also record heart rhythm.

What the results show. The test can detect irregular heartbeats and silent ischemia (periods when the heart muscle is not getting enough oxygen).

Advantages. This test can detect intermittent abnormalities that can be missed by an ordinary ECG. It also allows your doctor can get a picture of your heart activity as you go about your normal routine. The monitor is small enough to wear in a shoulder harness, in a pocket, or attached to your belt (see Figure 4).

Disadvantages. It may miss serious abnormalities that occur at times other than during the test. A lead may loosen or give misleading results if it gets wet.

EXERCISE ELECTROCARDIOGRAPHY (STRESS TEST)

ECG leads are attached to the chest and a blood pressure cuff is put in place. The patient then exercises on a treadmill or stationary bicycle while the heart rate, ECG pattern, and blood pressure are monitored during the exercise (Figure 5). The exercise intensity is generally increased every three minutes until the heart rate reaches a certain level or symptoms such as fatigue, chest pain, a drop in blood pressure, or dizziness develop. The ECG is monitored constantly and recorded at each stage of exercise and during recovery. ECG abnormalities may mean significant coronary artery disease. To obtain additional information, the

FIGURE 3 (*opposite*). (*a*) Normal resting electrocardiogram. This is an electrocardiogram, or ECG, from a patient who has a regular heart rhythm and no evidence of a heart attack. The numbers and letters above the ECG tracing refer to each of the twelve ECG leads, or wires, that are attached to the patient with adhesive pads during the test. The six tracings on the left are derived from leads placed on the arms and legs, while the six tracings on the right are derived from leads placed across the chest. The rhythm is regular and the ECG is normal for each lead. (*b*) Electrocardiogram showing atrial fibrillation. In this ECG, the rhythm is irregular when compared to the normal rhythm in Figure 3a. In addition, there are significant abnormalities in the configuration of the ECG consistent with additional heart abnormalities. (*c*) Electrocardiogram showing ventricular tachycardia. This electrocardiogram is from an individual with ventricular tachycardia, a very abnormal heart rhythm. If untreated, this arrhythmia may progress and lead to sudden cardiac death. The heart rate here is faster than noted in the other ECGs. In addition, the ECG signal is much wider, indicating that the activity originates from the ventricles.

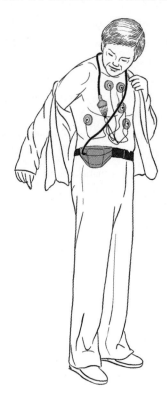

FIGURE 4. Holter monitor. When a Holter monitor is needed, ECG leads are attached to the chest and the portable monitor can be worn on a belt or carried in a pocket. The twenty-four-hour (or longer) recording is analyzed afterward.

exercise stress test may be combined with either nuclear (SPECT) or echocardiographic imaging (see later in this chapter).

What the results show. The test is done diagnostically to evaluate possible coronary artery disease and detect cardiac ischemia, periods when the heart muscle is not getting enough oxygen. Characteristic ECG changes occur during ischemia. This test is used to assess heart health following a heart attack, angioplasty, and coronary bypass surgery.

Advantages. The test provides a noninvasive method of assessing ECG changes that only occur under physical stress during vigorous exercise. It is generally safe when performed in the proper setting and under medical supervision and it can also help determine safe levels of exercise. It is relatively inexpensive.

Disadvantages. The results may often be unreliable; in fact, a significant por-

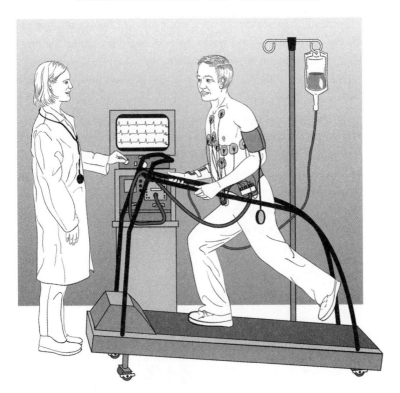

FIGURE 5. Exercise stress test. During an exercise stress test, electrocardiogram (ECG) leads, or wires, are attached to the patient's chest, and a blood pressure cuff is wrapped around an arm. An intravenous line is also inserted. The patient then exercises on a treadmill (or exercise cycle) under a doctor's or nurse's supervision until the target heart rate is reached or symptoms develop. The continuous ECG, with its multiple leads, is intended to detect coronary artery disease and other cardiac abnormalities.

tion of exercise stress tests may produce false-positive results. Such results are more common in women than men. The results also are often not sufficiently sensitive to detect significant coronary artery disease. In addition, many patients cannot achieve a significant enough rise in heart rate to achieve diagnostic accuracy.

RESTING ECHOCARDIOGRAPHY (CARDIAC ULTRASOUND)

In resting echocardiography, high-frequency sound waves are directed into the chest to create an image of the heart. A gel is applied to the chest to help conduct the sound waves and, while the patient lies quietly on an examination table, the person performing the test places over specific areas of the chest a transducer that emits high-frequency sound waves used to create images of the heart or other internal organs (Figure 6). In a variation called Doppler ultrasound, a special microphone is used to measure the velocity of blood flow in the heart or other blood vessels, especially the carotid arteries in the neck.

What the results show. Echocardiography provides images of the heart structures, thereby providing important information about various heart defects. It also measures the size of the heart and its chambers and helps evaluate the function of the heart muscle and valves (Figure 7). In addition, it can detect excessive fluid in the pericardium, the membrane that surrounds the heart.

Advantages. Echocardiography is painless, noninvasive, and safe, and the patient can resume normal activities immediately afterward.

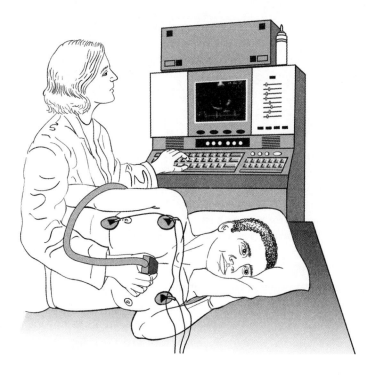

FIGURE 6. Resting echocardiography. While the patient lies on one side, a technician or physician creating a resting echocardiogram will pass an echo (sonar) transducer over the chest. The echoes created by the transducer create an image of the heart's structures; it can also measure blood flow through the heart, which will help identify and characterize leaky or narrowed heart valves.

NORMAL

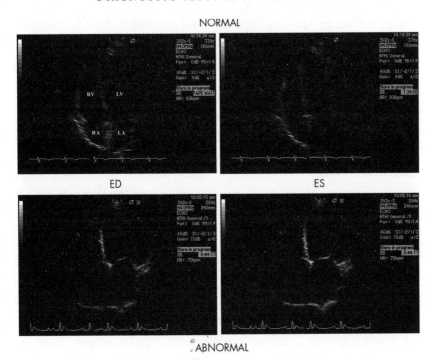

ABNORMAL

FIGURE 7. Echocardiograms of a normal and abnormal heart. Two isolated frames are shown. ED represents end diastole, when the heart is at its largest volume. ES represents end systole, when the heart is at its smallest volume. The echocardiogram in the upper left is labeled to indicate the cardiac structures visualized. The orientation is the same for all four echocardiograms. RV is the right ventricle, LV is the left ventricle, RA is the right atrium, and LA is the left atrium. In the top two pictures you can see how the heart volume decreases from ED to ES, indicating that the heart is pumping effectively. In the abnormal echocardiogram shown in the bottom two images, there are only minor changes from ED to ES, indicating that the patient's heart is functioning poorly.

Disadvantages. Chest-wall abnormalities and other diseases, such as emphysema, can distort the results.

EXERCISE (STRESS) ECHOCARDIOGRAPHY

Exercise echocardiography evaluates the heart before and after an exercise stress test. It uses the same techniques described in the sections on resting echocardiography and exercise electrocardiography. For people unable to exercise, the test can be done by administering a drug (dobutamine) to speed the heartbeat to adequate levels. The drug may be given at a lower dosage to test heart muscle viability, that is, to stimulate ischemic heart muscle that is functioning poorly but nevertheless is still alive.

What the results show. The test provides information about abnormal heart function that occurs during exercise but is not present when resting. This is an indication of abnormal blood flow (ischemia) and is used diagnostically.

Advantages. It is noninvasive and generally safe when done under proper medical supervision.

Disadvantages. As with exercise electrocardiography, the combined test can give false-positive and false-negative results.

NUCLEAR STRESS TEST

This noninvasive nuclear stress test uses a radioactive tracer to provide a three-dimensional view of the heart's muscle and blood flow through single photon emission computed tomography, or SPECT. It is often used to determine whether a patient should undergo additional, perhaps invasive, examinations such as cardiac catheterization. Following an exercise stress test (or administration of the drugs adenosine or dobutamine, for patients who cannot exercise), a radioactive substance is injected into the bloodstream and then rapidly taken up by the heart muscle in proportion to the blood flow to the heart. If a portion or portions of the heart do not receive enough blood due to narrowing of the coronary arteries, this will be detected as an area of decreased radioisotope uptake. A special instrument detects the radioactivity and constructs a "heart scan," or three-dimensional image of the heart (Figure 8). Studies obtained during stress and then again at rest are compared in order to identify the heart regions that are not receiving enough blood flow when it is needed.

What the results show. The test assesses the amount of blood reaching the heart muscle; it can identify specific areas of heart muscle that are not getting enough blood and consequently identify blocked or narrowed coronary arteries. It is also used to study the effectiveness of coronary bypass surgery or angioplasty, and can provide insight into the viability of particular areas of heart muscle.

Advantages. The test is noninvasive and provides clear three-dimensional pictures of the heart's structure and function. It provides a more accurate diagnostic picture in a woman than is generally obtained during an exercise stress test alone.

Disadvantages. There may be some mild discomfort when the intravenous line for radioisotope injection is initially placed. Some people, especially those

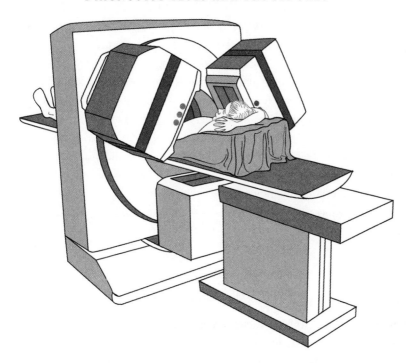

FIGURE 8. Imaging by a gamma camera as part of a nuclear stress test. In a nuclear stress test, special radioactive material is injected into the patient's circulation after the patient exercises. The radioactive material is taken up in the heart according to its blood flow. A gamma camera then records and constructs an image of the activity in the heart muscle in order to find any areas of the heart not receiving enough blood flow.

who suffer from claustrophobia, may also find it uncomfortable to lie under the SPECT camera for thirty to forty-five minutes. Obesity can result in poor images.

TRANSESOPHAGEAL ECHOCARDIOGRAPHY

Transesophageal echocardiography, or TEE, involves spraying the throat with a local anesthetic to reduce the gag reflex and then passing a hollow tube (an endoscope) containing a small transducer, similar to the ones used in echocardiography, down the esophagus. This allows the examiner to transmit high-frequency sound waves to the heart from inside the body, in order to create a detailed image. It is especially useful in diagnosing heart valve disorders and congenital heart disease and in providing information about the left atrium (the heart's major pumping chamber); for example, the presence of blood clots. It is also useful for detecting an aortic aneurysm dissection or rupture.

What the results show. The test provides images of the heart that may be difficult or impossible to obtain during conventional echocardiography. It can also be used to monitor heart function during cardiac surgery and to detect blood clots in the left atrium, the heart chamber that receives blood that has circulated through the body.

Advantages. TEE is especially useful in examining the heart in very obese patients or those who have unusually thick chest walls—obstacles that hinder conventional echocardiography.

Disadvantages. Insertion of the endoscope causes some discomfort and carries a slight risk of bleeding or, more rarely, perforation of the esophagus.

CARDIAC CATHETERIZATION AND CORONARY ANGIOGRAPHY

This two-part test, which involves cardiac catheterization and coronary angiography, is carried out in a hospital catheterization lab or special diagnostic center. It is used to evaluate coronary arteries and other heart structures by providing images and measurements that cannot be obtained through noninvasive studies. It is especially useful for evaluating patients with unstable angina, chest pains that occur even during rest. It is typically done on an outpatient basis unless the patient is already hospitalized. The patient is given a sedative and a small incision is made in a blood vessel, usually an artery in the leg or arm, and a thin catheter is passed through the vessel to the heart (catheterization). A contrast dye is then injected to make the coronary arteries and other heart structures visible on X-ray movies (angiography). (See Figure 9.) In a variation of the procedure called endomyocardial biopsy, tissue samples can be collected during cardiac catheterization to assess possible heart muscle disorders and are often used initially after heart transplantation to detect rejection.

What the results show. Cardiac catheterization and angiography can pinpoint narrowings and blockages in the coronary arteries; the test also allows doctors to evaluate the function of bypass grafts, the state of arteries beyond the area of blockage, heart valves, and other heart structures.

Advantages. The test provides images and information that cannot be obtained through less invasive examinations. Often angioplasty, a procedure to increase blood flow through the coronary arteries, and insertion of a stent to keep

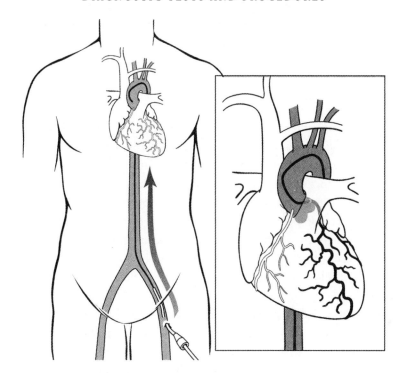

FIGURE **9**. Cardiac catheterization. During cardiac catheterization, a very small tube, called a catheter, is inserted into an artery (typically one in the groin as illustrated here) and then threaded through the arteries to the heart. Dye can then be injected through the catheter to make the coronary arteries (insert) visible as X-ray movies. Other heart structures can also be examined during the procedure.

the vessels open, can be carried out immediately after the examination. (See Chapter 7.) Intravascular ultrasound (IVUS) can also be done during the cardiac catheterization to provide even more information concerning specific areas of the coronary artery that cannot be evaluated definitively with angiography.

Disadvantages. This test is invasive and carries a small risk of bleeding at the site where the catheter is inserted; it may also promote formation of a blood clot. In very rare cases, a blood vessel may be punctured or the test may precipitate a heart attack, stroke, or cardiac arrest. Some people experience allergic reactions to the dye; be sure to tell your doctor if you are allergic to seafood or other substances containing iodine. If so, specific desensitization procedures can be carried out in advance to prevent an allergic reaction. In individuals with poor kidney function, the procedure can result in a further decline.

ELECTROPHYSIOLOGICAL TESTING

Electrophysiological testing (EPS), which is done in a hospital catheterization lab or diagnostic center, uses the same initial steps as cardiac catheterization. After the catheter reaches the heart, electrodes are guided into the heart to make detailed recordings of its electrical activity and pathways. When the electrodes are in place, drugs may be administered to study their effectiveness.

What the results show. The test can pinpoint areas of the heart muscle that are sending out or conducting abnormal electrical impulses, causing potentially serious cardiac arrhythmias. Sometimes it is done before insertion of a cardiac pacemaker or before an area of the heart causing a rhythm disturbance is ablated (destroyed).

Advantages. The test provides information that cannot be obtained through less invasive studies. And during the procedure, an abnormal electrical pathway may be made inactive (ablation).

Disadvantages. Beyond the risks of cardiac catheterization, which are also present in this test, it may provoke serious arrhythmias.

UPRIGHT TILT-TABLE TESTING

The tilt-table test helps diagnose patients who have a form of fainting called neurocardiogenic syncope, which is caused by interactions between the autonomic nervous system and the heart. Individuals lay flat on their backs on a tilt-table, then are tilted upright to a maximum of 60 to 80 degrees for twenty to forty-five minutes. In a positive test, the heart rate and blood pressure fall, often reproducing the symptoms the patient has experienced. At times, a drug (isoproterenol) is given during this test to increase the likelihood of an abnormal response.

What the results show. This test will identify two-thirds to three-quarters of all individuals who have neurocardiac causes for fainting.

Advantages. Because it provides highly reliable information concerning neural-mediated syncope, or fainting, a positive response can help lead to therapy to prevent the fainting episodes.

Disadvantages. The test may produce the patient's actual symptoms and lead to a fainting episode, but this can generally be rapidly reversed.

POSITRON-EMISSION TOMOGRAPHY

In the PET scan, radioactive substances (positron-emitting isotopes) are used to assess the viability of and blood flow to the heart muscle. After the isotopes are injected, the patient is positioned under a special tomographic camera, which creates a three-dimensional image of the heart and records the heart muscle's uptake of the radioactive substances.

What the results show. The test provides specific information about blood flow to the heart muscle and the muscle itself.

Advantages. The test is noninvasive and thus does not carry the risk of catheterization and other invasive examinations. It is more sensitive than SPECT or echocardiography and is better suited for obese patients.

Disadvantages. It is expensive and as yet, not widely available, although it is becoming more commonly used, especially for determining the stage (extent) of cancer.

COMPUTED TOMOGRAPHIC ANGIOGRAPHY

Computed tomographic angiography involves the intravenous injection of radiographic contrast material, which is then recorded in less than a minute by a highly sophisticated tomographic X-ray device that provides a three-dimensional reconstruction of images of the heart and blood vessels. This technique, which is still in its early stages, allows detection of diseases of the blood vessels (vasculature), such as an aortic aneurysm, and provides detailed images of your heart structures and coronary arteries. In certain instances, it provides noninvasive information similar to that obtained by coronary angiography.

What the results show. The images are often of very high resolution, providing information concerning the anatomy of the heart and blood vessels.

Advantages. In the future, this method of testing may provide a noninvasive means of detecting coronary artery narrowing that now requires coronary angiography. It can also provide relevant information on how bypass grafts are faring and whether an aneurysm has formed in the aorta or other blood vessels.

Disadvantages. This technique is still evolving and is expensive; it also administers a significant dosage of radiation to the patient. Intravenous medication is often required during the test.

COMPUTED TOMOGRAPHIC CALCIUM SCORING

Although atherosclerosis does not always produce calcium deposits within blood vessel walls, in a significant number of cases it does. Computed tomographic scanning allows visualization of this calcium in the coronary arteries, and can define the amount that is present as well as its location. The larger the amount of calcium, the greater is the risk of significant coronary atherosclerosis and a subsequent heart attack or other cardiac event.

What the results show. The calcium present in the coronary arteries is scored. A high score is associated with significant coronary atherosclerosis. An abnormal result would generally indicate a need for further tests, such as stress imaging studies or coronary angiography.

Advantages. This is a relatively simple test that can be done in a matter of minutes.

Disadvantages. The study only tells you about the presence of calcium and does not define whether the coronary arteries have any areas that are significantly narrowed. In addition, insurance generally does not cover the test.

MRI/MRA (MAGNETIC RESONANCE
IMAGING AND ANGIOGRAPHY)

Various components of human tissue have magnetic properties that are stimulated when they are placed in an external magnetic field. This expression results in the emission of a signal that can be detected by MRI/MRA and then translated into cross-sectional and three-dimensional images. A contrast material, when given intravenously, can enhance the visualization of blood vessels (angiography).

What the results show. MRI/MRA produces extremely high resolution images of the heart's anatomy and can also provide information on cardiac function. The test is also very useful in producing images of blood vessels, especially when contrast material is used, providing a noninvasive alternative to cardiac catheterization and angiography. The use of other agents may allow for detection of ischemia comparable to that obtained with stress echocardiography and stress SPECT studies.

Advantages. This is a noninvasive test that does not use radiation. The resolution is extremely high and thus provides detailed insight into cardiovascular anatomy not readily activated with other technology.

Disadvantages. In cardiovascular medicine, this technology is used predominately for research and is not yet widely available in clinical settings. It is also expensive. In general, it cannot be used in patients with implanted defibrillators and/or pacemakers.

PACEMAKER/IMPLANTED CARDIAC DEFIBRILLATOR FOLLOW-UP

Sometimes the functioning of an implanted cardiac pacemaker or implanted cardiac defibrillator (ICD) needs to be checked regularly. Such tests can be done in a doctor's office or testing center, or from home using special telephone monitoring equipment.

What the results show. The tests, which should be done on a regular basis, check the devices' signals and batteries to make sure they are working properly.

Advantages. Newer devices provide a record of activity and actually record rhythm disturbances, allowing a doctor to determine whether problems have occurred since the last follow-up.

Disadvantages. None.

ENDOTHELIAL FUNCTION TESTING

Recently it has become clear that the internal lining of blood vessels (the endothelium) is an active organ. Disorders in the endothelial lining of blood vessels occur early in the course of arteriosclerosis and provide an important indication of an early phase of blood-vessel disease. Normally, when a blood vessel is blocked and then opened, there is a substantial increase in blood flow through that vessel—a response mediated by the endothelium (hyperemic response). This response can be quantified, thereby providing a noninvasive means of detecting abnormal endothelial function. This increase of blood flow can be detected by placing an ultrasound probe over the arm's brachial artery or by using a finger cuff device (plethysmograph). The blood vessel is then closed by tightening a blood pressure cuff. When the cuff is loosened, there should be a measurable and predictable increase in blood flow; if this does not occur, it is a sign of endothelial dysfunction. Endothelial dysfunction observed in the arm or finger generally correlates with the same condition in the coronary arteries.

What the results show. The test allows definition of the hyperemic response, which signifies normal endothelial function.

Advantages. Because the endothelium generally functions the same throughout the body's circulatory system, abnormalities detected in the arm or finger correlate well with abnormalities in the coronary arteries. The tests are noninvasive and can be done relatively quickly.

Disadvantages. Until now, these techniques have been used mostly for research purposes; they are, however, likely to be available soon for clinical applications.

VASCULAR ULTRASOUND

Vascular ultrasound involves direct ultrasound imaging of blood vessels such as the carotid arteries in the neck, femoral arteries in the leg, and so forth. The ultrasound images help localize any narrowings. Addition of a Doppler technique allows the measurement of blood flow.

What the results show. The results define narrowings in peripheral blood vessels. It can also be used to detect an aortic aneurysm in the abdomen.

Advantages. The test is noninvasive and can be done relatively quickly.

Disadvantages. At times it may be difficult to define the exact areas of vessel abnormalities.

ANKLE/BRACHIAL INDEX

The ankle/brachial index (ABI) is the ratio of blood pressure in the arm (brachial) compared to that in the ankle. These pressures are measured with a Doppler ultrasound probe and a blood pressure cuff. The goal is to detect peripheral vascular disease in the lower extremities.

What the results show. If the difference between the blood pressure in the arm and the ankle is greater than 20 mm Hg, it indicates a blockage of the arteries of the legs. The test is also used to gauge the severity of the blockages.

Advantages. The test is noninvasive and it can be repeated as necessary without any adverse effects.

Disadvantages. The test is not reliable in individuals who have calcified vessels because these vessels cannot be compressed by the blood pressure cuff.

GENETIC TESTING

It is increasingly clear that a number of cardiovascular conditions are inherited and consequently may be detected by genetic testing. When an abnormal gene is identified, it may be possible to detect its presence, from either a simple blood test or a tissue biopsy.

What the results show. Results of genetic testing vary depending on the genetic disorder being considered, but a significant increment or an overt expression of an abnormal gene may be a marker of disease or high risk of one.

Advantages. Genetic testing can provide important insights for families and lead to important genetic counseling concerning transmission of the disease to other family members. It can also identify carriers of a disease, as well as those who may or may not be afflicted during their lifetime but can transmit the condition to their offspring.

Disadvantages. None.

SUMMING UP

Doctors now have a wide array of diagnostic tools to help them pinpoint the type and extent of cardiovascular disease. Some of these tests are invasive and must be done in a hospital laboratory or diagnostic clinic; others are noninvasive and can be carried out in a doctor's office. And more sensitive tests are under development, promising even more accurate diagnosis in the future.

7

Treating Your Heart Condition

reat advances in the medical treatment of heart disease now enable millions of Americans to lead longer, more productive lives than would have been possible just a few decades ago. Indeed, some forms of cardiovascular disease that were once common and claimed many lives are now rare or virtually nonexistent. Take malignant hypertension, the disease responsible for the stroke that killed President Franklin D. Roosevelt in 1945. At that time, there was no effective drug treatment for high blood pressure, which often progressed to heart and kidney failure or, as in the case of FDR, the highly lethal malignant hypertension that culminated in a fatal stroke. Rheumatic heart disease, another major killer of the past, is now rare in the United States and other developed countries, thanks to the widespread use of antibiotics to prevent or treat rheumatic fever.

Most of the forms of heart disease that are still with us are now eminently treatable with a vast array of medications, implanted pacemakers, and surgery and other interventional procedures that not only relieve debilitating symptoms, but also extend life. Some of these advances, especially those that involve medications, are now accepted components of lifelong treatment plans, along with the healthy lifestyle changes discussed earlier. This chapter presents a broad overview of the medical treatments for the most common forms of heart disease. Very often, the treatment goal involves prevention of the progression of heart disease. So if you are found to have what was once considered mild high blood pressure or borderline elevated blood cholesterol or high blood sugar levels, treatment at an early stage is designed to forestall the need for later more invasive or aggressive treatments.

HIGH BLOOD PRESSURE

High blood pressure, or hypertension as it is known medically, is by far our most common form of cardiovascular disease, affecting more than 65 million Americans. In simple terms, hypertension is defined as excessive pressure exerted on the artery walls as blood is pumped through the body's circulatory system. Picture the circulatory system as a tree. The aorta (the body's largest artery, which arises from the heart) is comparable to the tree's trunk. A network of smaller arteries branch off the aorta, much as limbs branch off of a tree trunk. These arteries divide into even smaller arteries, called arterioles, which can be likened to twigs. Capillaries, the body's smallest blood vessels, are comparable to leaves, carrying oxygen and other blood-borne nutrients to individual cells. The oxygen-depleted blood then flows back to the heart through a system of increasingly large veins.

As it travels through the body, blood does not flow in a steady stream, as water flows from an open faucet. Instead, it moves in spurts. With each heartbeat, a few ounces of blood are pumped out of the heart and into the branching arterial system. A certain amount of force, or pressure, is necessary to keep the blood moving until it reaches the microscopic capillaries. This pressure is determined by the arterioles, the smallest of the arteries. To increase blood pressure, the arterioles narrow, or constrict; to lower the pressure, the vessels open up, or dilate.

Under normal circumstances, blood pressure is constantly adjusted by a complex system of hormones and nerve sensors. It can vary greatly over the course of a day, rising and falling according to the body's needs. For example, blood pressure typically rises when you exercise or confront a stressful situation. Hormones, especially those released by the kidneys and the adrenal glands, instantaneously signal the need for increased blood flow. The heart beats faster and harder, pumping out more blood with each beat. The arterioles constrict to raise pressure and increase blood flow to the parts of the body needing the extra oxygen. In contrast, blood pressure falls when you are sitting quietly or sleeping, reflecting the body's reduced need. In addition, the brain also senses when blood pressure is too low and signals the kidneys and adrenal glands to secrete hormones to raise it.

High blood pressure occurs when the arterioles are chronically constricted. Over time, this increased pressure takes a toll on many parts of the body, especially the heart, brain, blood vessels, and kidneys. Thus, untreated high blood pressure greatly increases the risk of a heart attack, heart failure, stroke, and kidney failure. It also increases your chance of developing an aortic aneurysm, in which a weakened section of the artery balloons outward and eventually may rupture. Excessive blood pressure can also damage the tiny blood vessels in the eye and contribute to a loss of vision. The situation is complicated by the fact that high blood pressure does not produce symptoms until it reaches an advanced stage and has caused a stroke, heart attack, or kidney failure. This is why high blood pressure is often referred to as the silent killer.

Detecting High Blood Pressure

Blood pressure is expressed in two numbers, such as 120/80. The higher number, called the systolic pressure, represents the maximum pressure exerted against the arterial walls during the heartbeat. The lower number, the diastolic pressure, is the amount of pressure exerted when the heart momentarily rests between beats.

Blood pressure is measured by a sphygmomanometer (pronounced sfig-moe-man-OM-e-ter), which consists of an inflatable rubber cuff, an air pump, and a column of mercury, dial, or digital readout reflecting the pressure in an air column. Typically, the cuff is wrapped around the upper arm, and the cuff is tightened until blood flow through the large artery in the arm is cut off. The person measuring the blood pressure then places a stethoscope over the artery, and as the cuff is loosened, listens for the first thumping sound, which signals the resumption of blood flow through the artery, and notes the pressure at this instant. He or she then loosens the cuff even more, and listens for the cessation of the thumping sound, indicating the diastolic pressure. The pressure reading is expressed in millimeters of mercury, abbreviated as mmHg. The simplest blood pressure machines actually use a column of mercury; newer devices have a dial or digital readout and are automated: no one is required to listen with a stethoscope.

A diagnosis of high blood pressure cannot be based on a single reading; instead, several measurements taken at different times and in varying circumstances are needed to establish an accurate diagnosis (see Table 7.) For example, a doctor may measure blood pressure at the beginning of an examination, and again later in the visit. In any event, a carefully calibrated machine is used, with the patient seated and after five minutes of rest. Moderately elevated measurements will be rechecked at a later visit and subsequent visits. In general, consistent readings of 140/90 or higher constitute high blood pressure and warrant some form of treatment.

TABLE 7

DIAGNOSIS AND MANAGEMENT OF HIGH BLOOD PRESSURE

Classification	Systolic Blood Pressure (mm/Hg)		Diastolic Blood Pressure (mm/Hg)	Action
Normal	<120	and	<80	Recheck in 2 years
Prehypertension	120–139	or	80–89	Recheck in 1 year; lifestyle modification
Stage 1 Hypertension	140–159	or	90–99	Recheck in 2 months; lifestyle modification, drug therapy
Stage 2 Hypertension	> 160	or	> 100	Recheck in 1 month; likely will need at least 2 drugs to treat

Source: Adapted from "Seventh Report of the Joint National Committee on Prevention, Detection, Evaluation and Treatment of High Blood Pressure (JNC-7)," *Hypertension* 42 (2003): 1206.

Drug Treatments for High Blood Pressure

In most instances—perhaps as many as 95 percent of cases—there is no identifiable reason for the elevated blood pressure; this is referred to as essential hypertension. In relatively uncommon instances, hypertension may be caused by narrowing of the arteries supplying the kidneys or, less commonly, by tumors of the adrenal gland. Some people with stage 1 hypertension—for example, a systolic pressure that ranges between 140 and 159, and a diastolic pressure that spans 90 to 99—may be able to lower their blood pressure with lifestyle changes. (Many, if not most, however, will require medication.) These lifestyle changes include losing excess weight, increasing exercise, reducing salt intake, and controlling stress. Of these, weight loss is the most important lifestyle modification; it's also very important to restrict salt intake because sodium prompts the body to retain water, which in turn increases blood volume and the heart's workload and thus raises blood pressure in many people. African Americans and the elderly are especially salt-sensitive, and lowering salt intake is an important component of treating patients in these groups. (Persons with heart failure should also restrict their salt intake.) You can start reducing your salt intake by not using it when cooking and not putting a salt shaker on the table. Indeed, many people automatically reach for the salt shaker before even tasting a food and complain that unsalted food lacks flavor. Flavor can be enhanced by substituting various herbs, spices, and lemon. Remember, too, that most commercially prepared foods, especially canned soups and vegetables, are loaded with salt. Always check the labels for sodium content, and select items that are salt-free or at least low-salt. (See Chapter 3 for a more detailed discussion on reducing salt intake.)

Although lifestyle changes are important in controlling high blood pressure, in most instances drugs, called antihypertensive agents, are also needed. The choice of medication depends on many factors, including age, gender, race, and personal preferences and circumstances. Guidelines issued in 2003 indicate that diuretics—among the oldest and least expensive drugs used to treat high blood pressure—are often the most effective initial medication.

Some of the drugs used to treat high blood pressure are also used for other forms of cardiovascular disease. For example, if you have both high blood pressure and angina, a single drug may treat both problems. But very often—maybe in even the majority of hypertensive patients—several different drugs are needed to bring the blood pressure to the desired goal, and additional ones may be added over time. These additions are not a sign of treatment failure, but rather represent a fine-tuning to find the most effective regimen. In fact, a period of trial and error is often needed to find the right combination of medications for you. During this time, your doctor may ask you to monitor your blood pressure at home and keep a diary of the readings. Automated home blood pressure machines are available at pharmacies, medical supply stores, and other outlets. (See Box 15 for guidelines on measuring your own blood pressure.)

As with any medication, antihypertensives can cause a variety of side effects. Some of these fade with time, whereas others may become intolerable. It is very important to report any side effects to your doctor, who can usually come up with a different dosage or combination of drugs that minimize the problem. In any event, you should never stop taking an antihypertensive drug or alter the dosage without first consulting your doctor. Abruptly stopping a drug can result in rebound hypertension, in which the blood pressure soars to pretreatment levels or goes even higher.

Box 15

MONITORING YOUR OWN BLOOD PRESSURE

Many doctors advise patients to monitor their own blood pressure between visits. You can do this with a home blood pressure machine, which you can purchase at a pharmacy or medical supply shop. These highly automated devices are easy to use and display the blood pressure in a digital readout; most also record the pulse rate.

Before starting home monitoring, ask your doctor, pharmacist, or other health professional to show you how to do it properly. In addition, home monitoring machines should be checked periodically by a doctor or other health professional to make sure they are properly calibrated. (Note that the coin-operated blood pressure machines found in many supermarkets, airports, and pharmacies are often unreliable, and their use for self-monitoring generally is not recommended.)

Avoid drinking coffee, tea, colas, and other caffeinated beverages for at least thirty minutes before measuring your blood pressure because caffeine raises blood pressure. The same applies to nicotine, including nicotine gum. (Of course, if you smoke, you should make every effort to stop.)

When measuring your blood pressure, sit in a relaxed position, with your arm about level with your heart and resting on a table. If you get a very high or low reading, wait a few minutes and repeat. Contact your doctor if you consistently have a high reading (for example, 140/90) or have symptoms such as dizziness or light-headedness.

There are eight major classes of antihypertensive drugs that may be used in your treatment. We discuss them generally here; see Table 8 for examples of each.

Diuretics or Water Pills

Diuretics are the oldest of the antihypertensive drugs—the first ones were introduced in the 1950s—and they remain among the most widely prescribed, inexpensive, and highly effective medications used. They reduce blood pressure by prompting the body to excrete salt and excessive water, thereby reducing the volume of blood flowing through the arteries. They are often combined with other antihypertensives, and are most effective in older people; they are also more effective in African Americans than are some of the newer drugs.

Beta Blockers

Also among the older antihypertensives are beta blockers. Introduced in the 1960s and 1970s, they are also a mainstay in the treatment of angina and heart failure. They work through the body's autonomic (automatic) nervous system, which regulates the heartbeat and other involuntary functions. They block certain nerve receptors, resulting in a slowing of the heart rate, even during rest. They also reduce the amount of blood pumped during each heartbeat, and lower the amount of oxygen needed by the heart muscle. These drugs are especially useful in patients who have high stress levels as well as those who have angina.

ACE (Angiotensin Converting Enzyme) Inhibitors

ACE inhibitors, introduced in the 1980s, work by inhibiting the production of angiotensin II, a body chemical that constricts blood vessels and plays a central role in raising blood pressure. They are often prescribed along with a diuretic, and are especially effective in patients who also have congestive heart failure. They may also be prescribed for patients who have diabetes because they may help protect the kidneys from diabetes-related damage; in addition, they may be used to treat patients with congestive heart failure. They can cause a dry cough, however, which limits their use by some patients.

Angiotensin-Receptor Blockers

These drugs, introduced in the 1990s, also work by blocking angiotensin II downstream, but they have fewer adverse effects than do the ACE inhibitors, especially for patients who also have diabetes. They often work best when prescribed along with a diuretic.

Calcium Channel Blockers

Introduced in the 1970s and 1980s, calcium channel blockers work by blocking the entry of calcium into the muscle cells that control the artery walls. Because calcium is necessary in order for muscles to constrict, blocking the entry of some of this calcium relaxes the arterioles and lowers blood pressure. They are often effective drugs of choice for people who also have angina, and may be combined with a diuretic, ACE inhibitor, or other antihypertensive medication.

Vasodilators

These drugs, introduced in the 1950s, are among the older antihypertensives; they work by widening, or dilating, the arterioles. They are usually prescribed with other medications, such as a beta blocker or diuretic. They may also be given intravenously or by injection to rapidly lower blood pressure during a hypertensive crisis.

Alpha-Blocking Agents

Alpha-blockers work through the autonomic nervous system to block the nerve (alpha adrenergic) receptors that cause constriction of the arterioles. These drugs can cause a sudden drop in blood pressure when a person stands up quickly—a condition called orthostatic hypotension. Consequently, they are not prescribed very often, and when they are, they are usually reserved for patients whose blood pressures are not controlled with more common drugs or combinations. They may also be prescribed for men with high blood pressure and an abnormal urinary stream—usually due to prostate problems—because they treat both conditions.

Centrally Acting Drugs

The centrally acting drugs are older antihypertensive medications, introduced in the 1960s and 1970s, and are not prescribed very often. They reduce the number of nerve impulses coming from the brain, lowering the heart rate and dilating the arterioles. When prescribed, these drugs are usually given along with a diuretic.

Possible Interventions

In unusual circumstances, hypertension has a specific cause, such as a narrowed or constricted renal (kidney) artery or a tumor that produces large amounts of adrenal (stress) hormones. Tests are ordered if a doctor suspects that high blood pressure may have an identifiable physical cause. These may include ultrasound or computed tomography (CT) or magnetic resonance angiograms (MRA), tests in which scans are made after injection of a dye to make the blood vessels visible.

When a cause is diagnosed, an intervention may fully correct the underlying problem. For example, angioplasty and insertion of a stent or bypassing a blocked renal artery can cure hypertension caused by narrowing of this blood vessel.

TABLE 8

CLASSES OF ANTIHYPERTENSIVE MEDICATIONS

Class of medication (possible side effects)	Common examples by generic and brand name
Thiazide and related sulfonamide diuretics (Loss of potassium; impaired kidney function)	Chlorothiazide (Diuril); hydrochlorothiazide (Esidrix, Hydrodiuril, and others); indapamide (Lozol); and others
Loop diuretics (same as thiazides)	Bumetanide (Bumex); furosemide (Lasix); torsemide (Demadex)
Potassium-sparing diuretics (possible potassium buildup)	Amiloride (Midamor); eplerenone (Inspra); spironolactone (Aldactone); triamterene (Dyrenium)
Beta blockers (fatigue, cold extremities, dizziness, vivid dreams, sexual dysfunction)	Acebutolol (Sectral); atenolol (Tenormin); bisoprolol (Zebeta); metoprolol (Lopressor, Toprol); nadolol (Corgard); penbutolol (Levatol); pindolol; propranolol (Inderal); timolol (Blocadren); and others
ACE inhibitors (dry cough, impaired kidney function)	Captopril (Capoten); enalapril (Vasotec); lisinopril (Prinivil, Zestril); ramipril (Altace); and others
Angiotension receptor blockers (ARBs) (back pain and dizziness)	Losartan (Cozaar); valsartan (Diovan); candesartan (Atacand); telmisartan (Micardis); eprosartan (Teveten); olmesartan (Benicar)
Calcium channel blockers (some cause swelling of extremities, or "edema"; verapamil may cause constipation in some patients)	Amlodipine (Norvasc); diltiazem (Cardizem); nifedipine (Procardia, Adalat, and others); verapamil (Isoptin, Calan); and others
Vasodilators (dizziness when rising abruptly)	Hydralazine (Apresoline); minoxidil
Centrally acting alpha blockers (impaired concentration, sluggishness, dizziness)	Clonidine (Catapres); guanabenz (Wytensin); methyldopa (Aldomet)
Alpha blockers (general dizziness or dizziness when rising abruptly) (Note: These drugs are no longer frequently prescribed.)	Prazosin (Minipress); terazosin (Hytrin); doxasocin
Combined alpha and beta blockers (same as for alpha blockers)	Carvedilol (Coreg); labetalol
Peripheral-acting adrenergic antagonists (Note: These drugs are now seldom prescribed.)	Guanadrel (Hylorel); guanethidine (Ismelin); rauwolfia alkaloids (Raudixin); reserpine (Serpasil)

Similarly, the surgical removal of a hormone-producing tumor will cure the resulting hypertension.

Goals of Treatment

Doctors continue to debate just how much high blood pressure should be lowered. According to guidelines published in 2003, blood pressure should be less than 140/90 mmHg in otherwise healthy persons, and less than 130/80 mmHg for persons who have diabetes and/or kidney disease. The target blood pressure, however, may vary depending on individual circumstances.

In addition to reducing blood pressure to normal or near-normal levels, doctors also seek to devise a regimen that causes minimal adverse side effects. This often entails trying a number of combinations to find the most effective medications and dosages. Doctors also consider individual characteristics—age, race, gender, and coexisting diseases—in selecting medications (see Table 9).

CORONARY ARTERY DISEASE

The coronary arteries, which provide essential oxygen and nutrients to the heart muscle, are so named because they encircle the heart like a crown (see Figure 2 in Chapter 6). The body's entire volume of blood passes through the heart's chambers about every sixty seconds, but only a small portion of this—about 3 percent—is available to the heart muscle (the myocardium) itself.

Coronary artery disease, or CAD, develops when these coronary blood vessels become narrowed by a buildup of fatty plaque and/or calcium deposits, reducing the amount of blood available to the heart muscle. Typically, CAD is a gradual process that often begins early in life but does not cause obvious problems for many years. Over time, however, the arteries become increasingly clogged and stiffened—a process called atherosclerosis. This can result in ischemia—a condition in which the heart muscle itself does not get enough oxygen when needed, such as when you exercise or are under stress. A heart attack occurs when the affected artery becomes completely blocked, usually by formation of a blood clot (thrombus), resulting in damage to the heart muscle.

Detecting Coronary Artery Disease

All too often, the initial symptom is a heart attack or even cardiac arrest—the leading cause of sudden death. When symptoms do occur, they most commonly

TABLE 9

VARIABLES TO CONSIDER IN SELECTING ANTIHYPERTENSIVE MEDICATIONS

For African Americans	Calcium channel blockers and diuretics work best; ACE inhibitors, ARBs, and beta blockers can be made more effective by combining with a diuretic.
For those over age sixty	Calcium channel blockers and diuretics are often most effective; centrally acting drugs may cause or exacerbate depression; dosages may need to be adjusted to compensate for kidney or liver problems.
For those who have suffered a heart attack	Beta blockers protect against a recurrent heart attack.
For those who have high blood pressure and sexual dysfunction	Beta blockers and some diuretics may exacerbate the sexual problems; ACE inhibitors, ARBs, alpha blockers, calcium channel blockers, or vasodilators are better choices.
For those who have asthma or other chronic lung disorders	Avoid beta blockers: ACE inhibitors and diuretics are better choices.
For those who suffer from migraine headaches	Beta blockers or calcium channel blockers (such as verapamil and diltiazem) may help prevent the headaches in addition to treating the cardiovascular problem.
For those who also have episodes of rapid heartbeats (tachycardia)	A beta blocker or verapamil may be the drug of choice. Combining with a diuretic may be of further benefit.
For those who have a slow heartbeat	Avoid beta blockers, diltiazem, and verapamil.
For those who also have diabetes	ACE inhibitors may protect against kidney damage; alpha blockers are usually tolerated, but use beta blockers and potassium-sparing diuretics with caution.
For those who also have heart failure	ACE inhibitors or ARBs are often drugs of choice; beta blockers, diuretics, and vasodilators also have extra beneficial effects.
For those who also have kidney failure	Loop diuretics (bumetanide, furosemide, and metotazone) and vasodilators (minoxidil) may be drugs of choice. Use potassium-sparing diuretics and guanethidine with caution if at all.
For women who are pregnant	Methyldopa and labetalol are the drugs of choice; ACE inhibitors and ARBs are contraindicated in pregnancy; beta blockers may be used with caution. Diuretics are not first choice, but are probably safe.
For those with osteoporosis (bone thinning)	Potassium-sparing and thiazide diuretics may help preserve bones.
For those with a history of depression	ACE inhibitors, alpha blockers, diuretics, and guanethidine do not appear to worsen or provoke depression. Avoid centrally acting drugs (clonidine, methyldopa, and reserpine); beta blockers may also exacerbate the problem.
For those who also have gout	Avoid diuretics or use with caution as they can provoke an attack.
For those who also have Raynaud's phenomenon (blanching of the fingers or toes in cold weather)	Avoid beta blockers; instead, use ACE inhibitors, calcium channel blockers, diuretics, methyldopa, prazosin, or reserpine.

Source: Adapted from B. L. Zaret, M. Moser, and L. S. Cohen, eds., *Yale University School of Medicine Heart Book* (New York: Hearst Books, 1992).

involve chest pain (angina pectoris) and shortness of breath. Typically, these do not occur until the affected coronary artery is 50 to 70 percent narrowed, and by then the disease is in an advanced stage. Even at this stage, however, the person may not experience obvious symptoms, although the heart muscle is not getting enough oxygenated blood—a condition referred to as "silent ischemia." The presence and extent of CAD can be determined by a number of tests—including an ECG, exercise stress test with imaging, nuclear studies, echocardiography, and coronary angiography (see Chapter 6 for detailed descriptions of these tests).

Drug Treatments for Coronary Artery Disease

A number of variables influence the choice of treatment, including severity of symptoms, age, extent and nature of the coronary obstructions, risk factors, and coexistence of other disorders. Stable angina, which is often quite predictable because it develops at specific levels of physical exertion or other provocations, can usually be controlled by avoiding the triggering factors and/or taking antianginal medications, such as nitrates, beta blockers, or calcium channel blockers (see Table 10). Unstable angina, acute coronary syndrome (ACS), or acute myocardial infarction (MI), however, require urgent treatment that often involves surgery or another intervention. In addition, underlying causes or related conditions, such as high blood pressure, elevated blood cholesterol, or diabetes, will be treated. Aspirin is generally recommended as a way to help prevent the occurrence of blood clots in the coronary arteries.

Very often, patients take a combination of drugs, especially if they have multiple problems. So caution is needed to avoid potentially dangerous drug interactions. Follow-up blood tests are usually ordered to monitor for adverse reactions such as liver or kidney damage. In addition, over time the condition may change or the body may build a resistance to medications, requiring an adjustment in dosages or additional medications. Such medication adjustments are not signs that the treatment program is failing; instead, such changes are often needed to ensure maximum effectiveness.

Nondrug Treatments for Coronary Artery Disease

Unstable or progressively severe angina or heart attacks not controlled by medication often require interventions. The two major forms of intervention to treat acute or stable CAD are angioplasty and stent placement and coronary bypass surgery (newer and more experimental interventions are reviewed in Part IV).

TABLE 10

CATEGORIES OF MEDICATIONS FOR PATIENTS WITH CORONARY ARTERY
DISEASE AND ANGINA PECTORIS

Antianginal drugs by category (special cautions)	Examples
Nitrates (Note: *Nitrates should never be taken with drugs to treat erectile dysfunction, such as Viagra, because this combination may precipitously lower blood pressure and cause a heart attack, stroke, or serious arrhythmia.*)	Nitroglycerine tablets, spray, patches, and ointment; isosorbide mononitrate and dinitrate
Beta blockers	Propranolol, metropolol, atenolol, and many others
Calcium channel blockers	Diltiazem, amlopidine, verapamil, nifedipine, and others
Anticlotting drugs (anticoagulants, antiplatelet, and thrombolytic agents) (Note: *These drugs may cause excessive bleeding, so their use must be closely monitored.*)	Aspirin or acetylsalicylic acid (usually a baby aspirin or one-half of a regular aspirin); dipyridamole; warfarin (Coumadin); clopidogrel (Plavix); ticlopidine (Ticlid); guinolone derivatives (Cilostazol); heparin (including newly formulated Lovenox)

Angioplasty and Stents

Angioplasty and stent placement, which are part of a group of treatments called percutaneous coronary interventions (PCIs), are now popular alternatives to coronary bypass surgery and are the most common cardiac procedures performed. They are used quite widely throughout the world, both in stable patients and those acutely ill in the early hours of a heart attack. Angioplasty—the most widely used form of PCI—involves threading a balloon-tipped catheter through the coronary artery and then inflating the balloon at the site of blockage to flatten the fatty deposit and thereby widen the channel. Until about five or six years ago, the treated arteries experienced "restenosis" (that is, they re-narrowed) in about 40 percent of cases. To prevent restenosis, stents—tiny umbrella-like devices—are inserted into the artery to keep it open. Use of stents is now the rule. (See Figure 10 for an illustration of a stent.) Patients having the procedure generally stay in the hospital only overnight. PCI is being refined to improve its long-term results. For example, newer stents are impregnated with drugs that are slowly released over time to prevent clogging within the device itself.

Coronary Artery Bypass Surgery

Each year, more than 300,000 Americans, usually persons with severe blockages of more than one coronary artery, undergo coronary artery bypass graft surgery (CABG). Traditionally, the operation involves opening the chest to expose the heart, which is then temporarily stopped while a heart-lung machine is used to maintain vital circulation during the surgery. With the body temperature lowered to reduce metabolic needs, the surgeon attaches grafts to the coronary arteries to bypass the blocked areas. The grafts are usually taken from arteries in the wrist, from arteries elsewhere in the chest (the mammary arteries), or from a vein in the leg. After the grafts are in place and have been tested to make sure they are open (patent), the surgeon disconnects the heart-lung machine and administers an electrical shock to restart the heartbeat. The chest is then closed and the patient's body temperature is raised to normal levels. Immediately following the operation, the patient will be taken to an intensive care unit to be monitored for any complications. After a day or so, most patients can be weaned off the ventilator, which is used to assist in breathing, and taken to a coronary care unit to recover. Most leave the hospital after five or six days to continue recuperating at home. Cardiac rehabilitation generally begins five or six weeks later.

Over the last thirty years, there have been tremendous advances in coronary bypass surgery. Today, a significant portion of operations use minimally invasive techniques, which are performed without stopping the heart and using the heart-lung machine. This "off-pump" variation of the operation also can be performed through a small "keyhole" opening as well as through the more usual incision through the breastbone (sternum). Off-pump procedures reduce the risk of postoperative mental and kidney problems and are especially suitable for patients who also have cerebral vascular and/or kidney disease. They are also less traumatic and often allow the patient to recover more quickly than after traditional open-heart surgery using a heart-lung machine.

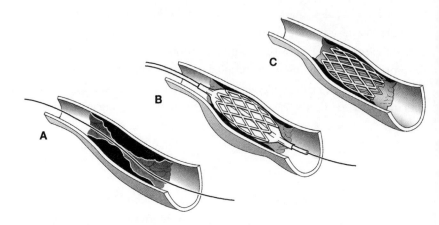

FIGURE 10. Balloon angioplasty and stent. To increase blood flow through a narrowed artery, a wire (A) is passed into the artery and a balloon-tipped catheter is placed over it. The balloon is inflated at the site of narrowing (B). This flattens the fatty deposits, thereby widening the channel. To keep the artery from renarrowing, a stent (C) is then permanently placed at the site of dilation.

Goals of Treatment

Treatment of coronary artery disease aims to eliminate or minimize symptoms as well as halt or minimize its progression. Angioplasty, bypass surgery, and other interventions can prevent or halt a heart attack. Sometimes treatment minimizes or even reverses damage from a heart attack. In any event, the overriding goal involves restoring the patient's ability to lead a normal, productive life.

ELEVATED BLOOD CHOLESTEROL

Cholesterol is a lipid, a fatty substance that circulates in the blood and is essential to maintaining the life of all animals, including humans. Meat, milk, eggs, and other animal products contain varying amounts of cholesterol, but it is not an essential dietary component because the body can make all that it needs. In humans, cholesterol serves three primary functions: it is essential to maintain cell membranes and structures; it is used to manufacture certain hormones, especially steroids and sex hormones; and the liver uses it to produce bile acids. Problems arise when too much cholesterol circulates in the blood and forms fatty deposits in the coronary arteries and other blood vessels.

Cholesterol travels through the blood attached to molecules called lipoproteins. The density of these lipoproteins determines whether cholesterol is potentially harmful or beneficial. Low-density lipoproteins are the most abundant, forming LDL cholesterol; this is often referred to as the "bad" cholesterol because excessive amounts tend to build up in the blood vessels. In contrast, high-density lipoproteins, which form HDL cholesterol, remove the fatty substance from the artery walls and carry it to the liver for excretion. Thus high levels of LDL cholesterol increase the risk of coronary artery disease, whereas high levels of HDL cholesterol lower risk.

Detecting High Cholesterol

Simple blood tests detect high blood cholesterol; these tests measure total cholesterol as well as the portions of HDL and LDL cholesterol. Levels of triglycerides, another blood lipid that may play a role in coronary artery disease, are also usually measured. About 25 percent of Americans have elevated cholesterol levels, generally defined as a total cholesterol reading of more than 200. Perhaps more telling, however, is the ratio of HDL to LDL cholesterol. For example, if you have a total cholesterol of 210, and your HDL level is 60 or higher, your risk is probably lower than someone whose total cholesterol is lower, but has an HDL level lower than 30.

Drug Treatments for High Cholesterol

Treatment for high cholesterol varies according to individual circumstances. Because cholesterol tends to rise with advancing age, an elderly person whose cholesterol is 220, for example, may not be treated as aggressively as would be a person in their thirties or forties who had comparable cholesterol readings. A healthy diet that is low in fat and cholesterol and high in fiber, as well as increased exercise, may be all that is needed to treat a person who has no other cardiovascular risk factors and only mildly elevated cholesterol. In contrast, aggressive drug treatment is recommended for patients with diagnosed heart disease or multiple risk factors. If you have significantly elevated cholesterol, diet alone is unlikely to be enough to treat it. Statins are the most effective cholesterol-lowering medications; these are usually recommended first. But there are alternatives for patients who cannot tolerate statins; see Table 11 for other medications your doctor might prescribe.

Goals of Treatment

In general, treatment is aimed at lowering LDL cholesterol and raising HDL levels. The target levels vary according to individual circumstances; for example, an LDL goal of 100 or less is recommended for persons with established heart disease or multiple risk factors. When risk is very high—defined as established heart disease plus multiple risk factors (smoking, metabolic syndrome, and acute coronary syndrome)—the LDL goal is 70 to 80 or lower.

HEART FAILURE

The term heart failure is something of a misnomer because it implies that the heart has ceased to function. Instead, it means that the heart is not pumping as efficiently as it should and, consequently, is failing to deliver adequate amounts of oxygen and other nutrients throughout the body. Heart failure afflicts about 5 million Americans, with more than 500,000 new cases diagnosed each year. In fact, heart failure is the single most common cardiovascular cause of hospital admissions in patients over age sixty-five in the United States.

Heart failure can occur at any age, but is most common among older people. Most often it results from damage of the heart muscle due to a heart attack, especially repeated attacks. Other possible causes include coronary artery disease, high blood pressure, defective heart valves, intrinsic disease of the heart muscle that has no known cause (cardiomyopathy), congenital heart defects, and infection or disease of the heart muscle. Some forms of heart failure are associated with pregnancy (peripartum cardiomyopathy); these often abate after delivery but they can cause severe problems for both mother and baby around the time of birth. Other conditions that contribute to heart failure include diabetes, anemia, excessive consumption of alcohol, viral infection (myocarditis), severe lung disease, cardiac arrhythmias, and an overactive thyroid (hyperthyroidism). Lifestyle factors—obesity and smoking, among others—can be contributing factors.

In addition to heart failure caused by heart muscle loss, there is another type associated with increasing heart muscle stiffness. This form, called diastolic heart failure, is especially common among the elderly. Heart failure also can result from excessive stiffness because of increased muscle in the heart from a type of cardiomyopathy called hypertrophic cardiomyopathy (HCM) or idiopathic hypertrophic subaortic stenosis (IHSS). Despite the different causes, the symptoms are identical.

TABLE 11

CATEGORIES OF LIPID-LOWERING MEDICATIONS

Drug category (special cautions)	Examples
Statins (Note: *These drugs sometimes cause muscle damage, so any muscle aches should be reported to your doctor.*)	atorvastatin (Lipitor); fluvastatin (Lescol); lovastatin (Mevacor); pravastatin (Pravachol); rosuvastatin (Crestor); simvastatin (Zocor)
Drugs that inhibit bile acid absorption	cholestyramine (Questran); colestipol (Colestid); colesevelam (WelChol)
Drugs that inhibit cholesterol absorption	ezetimibe (Zetia or Ezetrol)
Drugs to lower triglycerides (Note: *These drugs should be avoided or used with caution by persons also taking statins.*)	fenofibrate (Tricor); gemfibrozil (Lopid)
Miscellaneous other lipid-lowering drugs (Note: *These drugs should be used with great caution by persons with diabetes or glucose intolerance.*)	Niacin or nicotinic acid

In its early stages, heart failure often does not produce symptoms. For a time, the heart can compensate for its declining ability to pump by increasing its size and raising the heart rate to circulate the same amount of blood. In time, however, these compensatory measures fall short; the enlarged heart muscle further weakens and the heart cannot adequately empty with each beat. Excessive fatigue and shortness of breath, especially when climbing stairs or carrying a heavy package, are common early symptoms. Excess fluid may back up into the lungs and add to difficulty breathing and fatigue. Patients with heart failure often have difficulty breathing when lying flat, and will resort to sleeping propped up with several pillows or even sitting up in a chair. Fluid may also accumulate in other body tissue, especially the feet, ankles, and legs; in very advanced cases, it may also build up in the abdomen. In addition to obvious swelling, patients often notice an abrupt unexplained weight gain, or their shoes feel abnormally tight. Some may also notice palpitations or arrhythmias, either because the heart beats more rapidly in an attempt to pump out more blood or actually develops a rhythm disturbance. In its advanced stages, heart failure can cause mental changes, such as memory loss, confusion, or feelings of disorientation. Death is generally due to either pump failure or an arrhythmia affecting the left ventricle, the heart's main pumping chamber. (For a description of different levels of heart failure, see Box 16.)

Detecting Heart Failure

The diagnostic process typically starts with your doctor carefully listening to the heart and lung sounds through a stethoscope and looking for physical signs, such as swelling of the feet, ankles, or abdomen and a bluish skin color. If your doctor suspects heart failure, a number of diagnostic tests will be ordered. These typically start with an electrocardiogram to define the heart rhythm and detect other abnormalities and a chest X-ray to determine whether the heart is enlarged.

The heart's ejection fraction—the amount of blood that is pumped into the circulation with each heartbeat—will be measured. (Normally, half to two-thirds of the blood in the heart's left ventricle is forced into the aorta during each heartbeat.) This information is obtained generally by echocardiography, but also by equilibrium radionuclide angiocardiography (ERNA) scanning. These tests also allow a doctor to measure the thickness of the heart muscle, observe how well the heart is beating, and pinpoint the source of the problem (for example, a thickening of the left ventricle or a defective heart valve). Other possible tests include cardiac catheterization and angiography, exercise stress testing with imaging, and blood studies.

Drug Treatments for Heart Failure

There is no cure for most forms of heart failure, but an increasing number of patients are living longer, more comfortable lives. Treatments usually entail taking medication and making lifestyle changes that ease the heart's workload. In fact, most heart-failure patients take a combination of medications that are designed to lighten the load on the heart and strengthen its pumping action. Many of these drugs are used to treat other forms of heart disease, so an individual's regimen must be tailored to meet individual needs. Table 12 provides a more complete list of drugs used; here we describe some of the categories of medications that may be prescribed for you. Note that although most medications will be taken at home, in advanced cases it may be possible to regularly administer medications intravenously on an outpatient basis. Such outpatient centers are now being set up in the United States to deliver this "infusion therapy," with encouraging initial results.

Box 16

CLASSIFICATION OF HEART FAILURE

In general, heart failure is divided into four categories or classes, based upon the severity of a patient's symptoms. The one most commonly used is the New York Heart Association Functional Classification.

- *Class I.* No symptoms and no limitation in ordinary physical activity.
- *Class II.* Mild symptoms and slight limitation of ordinary activity; no symptoms when resting.
- *Class III.* Marked limitation in activity, even during less-than-ordinary activity; comfortable only when resting.
- *Class IV.* Severe limitations and symptoms (for example, shortness of breath) even when resting.

Diuretics

Diuretics lighten the heart's workload by prompting the kidneys to increase secretion of sodium and fluid, thereby reducing blood volume.

Nitrates

Used to treat angina, nitrates will also reduce filling pressures in the heart and can improve symptoms of heart failure.

Vasodilators

Vasodilators are also a mainstay in controlling high blood pressure. They work by dilating or widening the small peripheral arteries, thereby promoting increased blood flow to body tissues and making it easier for the heart to work. Vasodilators include ACE inhibitors and angiotensin receptor blockers (ARBs).

Beta Blockers

The beta blockers, which are also used to treat hypertension, a rapid heartbeat, and angina, work by decreasing the heart's workload and slowing the heart rate. Only a few years ago, beta blockers were considered potentially dangerous for heart-failure patients. But evidence now indicates that they are an extremely important part of therapy for heart failure. (See the drug section and tables in the hypertension section for a more detailed discussion and listing of specific drugs in each category.)

Alderosterone Blockers

By altering the effects of alderosterone, a hormone released by the adrenal gland, alderosterone blockers have been shown to improve symptoms of heart failure.

Digitalis

Originally derived from the foxglove plant, digitalis has been used since the eighteenth century, making it one of the oldest of all heart medications. It has been upstaged substantially by newer, more effective and safer drugs and is used infrequently at the present time. Nevertheless, it is still prescribed occasionally. It works by strengthening the heart's pumping action; it will also slow the heart rate in patients with atrial fibrillation.

Surgical Treatments for Heart Failure

In the last decade, advances in surgical treatment and interventional procedures have given new hope to many patients with even very advanced heart failure. The choice of procedure varies according to the cause and nature of the disease. Some patients undergo coronary bypass surgery and/or angioplasty—these operations, which increase blood flow to the heart muscle, are especially beneficial for patients whose heart failure is linked to coronary artery disease or damage from a heart attack. Other patients, particularly those whose heart failure stems from a defective or damaged heart valve, may benefit from heart-valve repair or replacement. Still other patients may be best served by new treatments discussed more fully in Chapter 15, including surgery to restore the shape of the ventricles, implanted defibrillators, resynchronization of the heartbeat, and ventricular assist devices.

Transplantation may be needed for some heart-failure patients, although it often remains as a last resort for the most seriously ill. The operation is often very successful: it is performed in many centers throughout the country, with a one-year survival rate of more than 85 percent. The major problem with transplantation remains the availability of donor hearts. In the year 2003, only 2,057

TABLE 12

CLASSES OF HEART FAILURE MEDICATIONS

Category	Examples
Diuretics	Furosemide, bumetanide, ethacrynic acid, hydrochlorothiazide, and others
Aldosterone blockers	Spironolactone, eplerenone
Nitrates	Isosorbide dinitrate and mononitrate
Vasodilators	Hydralazine
Angiotensin-converting enzyme (ACE) inhibitors	Captopril enalapril, lisinopril, ramipril, quinapril, and others
Angiotensin receptor blockers (ARBs)	Losartan, valsartan, candesartan, telmisartan, eprosartan
Beta-blocking agents	Metoprolol, bisoprolol, carvedilol
Digitalis	Digoxin
Natriuretic peptides	Nesiritide (given intravenously)

heart transplants were performed in the United States, which meant that only a small fraction of the number of patients on waiting lists were able to receive a donor heart that year.

Lifestyle factors are also key in treating heart failure. Salt restriction is especially important in helping prevent a buildup of body fluids. If you smoke, you should quit as soon as possible. Losing excess weight, limiting caffeine intake if you have heart-rhythm problems, consuming alcohol only in moderation, and reducing stress are also advisable. It's also important to control contributing disorders: in particular, you will want to lower high blood pressure, manage diabetes, and control high blood cholesterol.

Exercise can help improve the quality of life for heart failure patients. Despite severe impairment in heart function, most patients can still exercise regularly and significantly improve their endurance and fitness through training. Any exercise, however, must be undertaken with a doctor's guidance. Many doctors recommend participating in a medically supervised cardiac rehabilitation program, and a number of insurance and managed care plans now cover exercise rehabilitation for heart failure.

Goals of Treatment

Because most forms of heart failure cannot be cured, treatment is aimed at minimizing symptoms and prolonging life.

CARDIAC ARRHYTHMIA

Under normal circumstances, the adult heart beats sixty to one hundred times a minute, but this varies greatly from person to person as well as from one activity to another. The heart rate often falls with advancing age. Persons who have undergone exercise conditioning often have a normal resting heart rate of forty-five to fifty-five beats per minute, whereas a sedentary individual usually has a higher rate. This is because exercise conditioning increases the efficiency of the muscles in extracting oxygen from the blood. As you would expect, the heart beats faster whenever extra demands are placed on it. When you are sleeping or sitting quietly, your heart beats more slowly than when you are exercising or under stress.

A series of synchronized electrical impulses control the heartbeat. The impulses arise in the heart's pacemaker, or sinus node, a cluster of specialized cells located at the top of the right atrium. These electrical impulses stimulate the muscle tissue of the heart's upper chambers, the left and right atria, causing them to contract. The electrical impulses then travel to the atrioventrical (AV) node, which is located at the top of the wall of tissue (septum) between the right and left ventricles, the heart's major pumping chambers, and then to conducting fibers, called the His-Purkinje system, which direct the impulses to the bottom and then up the sides of the ventricles. This flow of electrical impulses results in coordinated contractions of the heart's chambers, allowing blood to be pumped from one part to another in an orderly fashion. All of this happens automatically, with various nerve impulses and hormonal signals instantaneously adjusting the heart rate.

Most people are unaware of their heart's beating, but from time to time, many experience palpitations, which may be felt as skipped beats, thumping, racing, or a fluttering sensation. You may be especially aware of palpitations before going to sleep, especially if you lie on your left side. This often happens because the sounds and distractions that normally mask the heartbeat are absent, and the bed may act like a drum, amplifying the sounds. Most palpitations are harmless, but those that cause symptoms—for example, light-headedness, dizziness, or fainting—may signal a cardiac arrhythmia.

There are two major types of cardiac arrhythmias: bradyarrhythmias, an abnormally slow heart rhythm of less than fifty-five or sixty beats a minute, and tachyarrhythmias, generally defined as a sustained rate of more than one hundred beats per minute. (Table 13 lists the various types of arrhythmias.)

Symptoms of a cardiac arrhythmia vary greatly and sometimes do not correlate with the severity of the underlying rhythm disorder. For example, some people with a serious arrhythmia may be unaware of any symptoms, while others with the same type of problem experience dizziness, fainting (syncope), and other symptoms. By the same token, some people who have a relatively benign condition may experience the same kind of troubling symptoms. Older people who have other forms of cardiovascular disease are more likely to experience symptoms than a young, generally healthy person. When symptoms occur, they may include:

- ♥ Dizziness, light-headedness, and unexplained fainting (syncope), which may occur with both slow and fast heartbeats.
- ♥ Chest pain and shortness of breath, which may occur when a very rapid heartbeat prevents the heart muscle from getting enough oxygen.
- ♥ Uncomfortable sensations, including pulsating, thumping, fluttering, or pounding.

Detecting Cardiac Arrhythmias

Most cardiac arrhythmias can be detected by an electrocardiogram (ECG or EKG). The various arrhythmias produce characteristic ECG tracings. A Holter monitor—a device that produces a continuous ECG over a period of twenty-four hours or longer—may be ordered to detect arrhythmias that occur only sporadically (see Chapter 6). Transtelephonic ECGs allow patients to record episodes of irregular heartbeats and transmit the ECG to a doctor via a telephone.

Electrophysiology studies are among the most sophisticated diagnostic and therapeutic techniques. During this procedure, an electrophysiologist threads several catheters containing electrodes through the venous system into the heart, and then makes detailed recordings of the heart's electrical activity. These studies are usually reserved for patients who are experiencing symptoms or those in whom a diagnosis is unclear. In patients whose rhythm disturbance can be treated with ablation—a procedure in which the defective electrical conduction cells are destroyed—the diagnostic study often will be done together with the treatment.

TABLE 13

TYPES OF CARDIAC ARRHYTHMIAS

Arrhythmia	Characteristics
Bradyarrhythmias	
Sinus bradycardia	Heartbeat slower than sixty beats per minute, originating in a malfunction of the sinus node
Sick sinus syndrome	Failure of the sinus node to conduct electrical impulses properly, usually causing a slow beat known as sinus bradycardia, which is also often associated with intermittent tachycardia—a fast heartbeat.
Heart block	Malfunction (block) of electrical system between the atria and ventricles, resulting in a very slow heart rate.
Tachyarrhythmias	
Supraventricular tachycardia	Rapid heartbeats arising in the atria or atrioventricular node, generally between 140 and 250 beats per minute.
Atrial flutter	"Circus current" due to an extra or premature beat that travels in cycles around the atrium, resulting in up to 300 atrial beats per minute
Atrial fibrillation	Chaotic, uncoordinated atrial beats of more than 350 beats per minute, resulting in a quivering of the atria. (It can also result in both rapid and slow heart rates.) It is most common in older people who have some other form of heart disease or, less commonly, thyroid disease (hyperthyroidism).
Wolff-Parkinson-White syndrome	Recurrent tachycardia caused by an abnormal conduction pathway, which in turn results in electrical impulses bypassing the atrioventricular node
Premature ventricular contractions (PVCs)	Early or extra beats that are often benign in a healthy heart but may be a harbinger of more serious, even lethal, episodes of ventricular fibrillation in persons with other heart disorders
Ventricular tachycardia	Abnormally rapid heartbeats that arise in the ventricles; can cause fainting (syncope) or lead to ventricular fibrillation
Ventricular fibrillation	Most severe form of ventricular tachyarrhythmia, in which the ventricles quiver at a very rapid rate and cease to pump blood; will cause death within minutes if the fibrillation is not reversed

Drug Treatments for Cardiac Arrhythmias

Treatment varies according to the specific type of arrhythmia, but it often involves a combination of interventions to restore a normal heartbeat, and then the use of antiarrhythmic drugs or a device to maintain it. (See Table 14.) Specific therapies include antiarrhythmic drugs, which are classified according to their mechanisms of action. For example, beta blockers (propranolol, timolol, and others) or calcium channel blockers (such as verapamil or diltiazem) may be prescribed to slow the rapid heartbeat of atrial fibrillation. Others, including sotalol and amiodarone, work by blocking potassium channels.

Another medical treatment employs anticoagulant drugs such as heparin and warfarin to reduce the buildup of blood clots. Such drugs are often prescribed in the treatment for patients with atrial fibrillation, a type of arrhythmia that can cause a pooling of blood in the heart's upper chambers (atria) and result in a blood clot. This sort of clot greatly increases the risk of an embolic stroke or other embolism.

Implanted Devices

Implanted devices can also be used to regulate the heartbeat. Pacemakers, for example, are a mainstay of treatment for abnormally slow heartbeats and may also be used to treat erratic arrhythmias. Implanted defibrillators are relatively new devices that are now widely used to prevent recurrent episodes of ventricular fibrillation in patients who have survived a cardiac arrest. They are programmed to detect the abnormal heartbeats and to administer an electrical shock to halt the fibrillation and restore normal rhythm. (Defibrillators are discussed in more detail in Chapter 15.)

Interventional Treatments

Some cardiac arrhythmias can be cured by surgery and other interventions. In one interventional procedure, called radiofrequency catheter ablation, a doctor threads a catheter through the blood vessels until it reaches the area of the heart muscle where the abnormal electrical pathway is located. A special probe applies a very high-frequency alternating current to destroy, or ablate, a small bit of heart muscle, thereby preventing the transmission of abnormal electrical impulses that cause erratic rapid heartbeats. The procedure is virtually painless and requires only mild sedation and local anesthesia. Patients can usually return to

TABLE 14

COMMON CARDIAC ARRHYTHMIAS AND CHOICES OF TREATMENT

Type of Arrhythmia	Treatment
Atrial fibrillation	*Acute:* cardioversion, ibulitide, flecainide, amiodarone, procainamide, beta blocker
	Long-term: beta blocker, sotalol, amiodarone, flecainide, procainamide, dofetilide, propafenone, aspirin or warfarin for anticoagulation, ablation
Atrial flutter	*Acute treatment:* cardioversion
	Long-term: verapamil, digitalis, amiodarone, ablation
Atrial premature complexes (APCs)	Generally, none. If symptomatic or precipitates tachycardia, a beta blocker or digitalis may be prescribed.
Atrial tachycardia	*Acute:* beta blocker, certain calcium channel blockers (verapamil and diltiazem), cardioversion
	Long-term: ablation, digitalis, beta blocker, calcium channel blocker, procainamide, flecainide, amiodarone
AV junction (AV node) tachycardia	*Acute:* adenosine, cardioversion, beta blockers
	Long-term: ablation, digitalis, beta blockers
Heart block	Insertion of a pacemaker
Sinus bradycardia (sick sinus syndrome)	Insertion of a pacemaker (if symptomatic)
Ventricular premature complexes (vpcs)	No treatment needed in absence of structural heart disease or symptoms; in such cases, beta blockers may be prescribed.
Ventricular tachycardia	*Acute:* cardioversion
	Long-term: ICD, amiodarone, sotalol, procainamide, mexiletine, flecainide

Note: *In many arrhythmias there are a number of drug options. Also, there are associated medical conditions that are beyond the scope of this overview, in which one treatment is favored over another. This must be discussed with your cardiologist. There are also special serious conditions associated with arrhythmias, such as Wolf-Parkinson-White syndrome, Long QT syndrome, and Brugada syndrome, which are not included in this listing.*

normal activities in a few days. More complicated ablation procedures are necessary for atrial fibrillation (see Chapter 15).

Goals of Treatment

Treatment is aimed at controlling the arrhythmia or its effects.

HEART-VALVE DISEASE

As blood is pumped through the heart's four chambers, it passes through a series of valves that open and shut to keep it moving in the right direction. Blood that has circulated through the body flows into the right atrium, which contracts to pump it through the tricuspid valve and into the right ventricle, one of the heart's lower pumping chambers. The blood is then pumped from the right ventricle through the pulmonary, or pulmonic, valve, into the pulmonary artery, and into the lungs where carbon dioxide is exchanged for a fresh supply of oxygen. The freshly oxygenated blood then flows back into the heart's left atrium and passes through the mitral valve into the left ventricle, the heart's main pumping chamber. As the left ventricle contracts, blood is forced through the aortic valve and into the aorta to begin another trip through the body's circulatory system (see Figure 2 in Chapter 6).

To control the flow of blood and ensure that it moves in the right direction, each chamber has a valve equipped with thin flaps of tissue, called leaflets or cusps, whose opening and closing determine the proper flow of blood. For example, the tricuspid valve has three leaflets and the mitral valve has two; the leaflets are connected to the muscle wall by chords of strong fibrous tissue called chordae tendineae. When open, the leaflets form a funnel-shaped ring that allows blood to pass through the valve; the leaflets then snap shut to prevent a backflow of blood.

The aortic and pulmonary valves are constructed somewhat differently. Instead of chords, they have petal-like flaps of tissue at their respective chamber exits. During each heartbeat, the petals open and then fall back together to close after blood passes through the valves.

Any defect or malfunction of these tiny structures is referred to as heart-valve disease (see Table 15 for common types). There are two major forms of heart-valve disease. In valvular stenosis, the heart valve fails to open properly and is generally quite narrowed, thereby preventing adequate amounts of blood from flowing from one part of the cardiovascular system to another. The stenosis may

TABLE 15

COMMON TYPES OF HEART-VALVE DISEASE

Disorder	Characteristics	Possible Treatments
Mitral valve prolapse (MVP)	The most common valvular disorder; it is marked by a deformity of the mitral valve in which leaflets fail to close properly. It is believed to be hereditary and is more common in women than men. It usually does not cause symptoms, but in some cases, may result in palpitation, chest pain, fatigue, shortness of breath, and fainting.	Usually does not require treatment unless it is causing symptoms. Medications, such as beta blockers, may be prescribed to slow a rapid heartbeat. In unusual cases, surgical valve repair/replacement may be needed. If mitral regurgitation is present, endocarditis prophylaxis should be used.
Mitral stenosis	A disorder in which the mitral valve stiffens or narrows, reducing blood flow to the left ventricle. It may eventually lead to heart failure; it can also cause atrial fibrillation.	It may be treated with surgical repair (commissurotomy), or in severe cases, valve replacement. Drugs may be prescribed to treat symptoms.
Mitral regurgitation	A disorder in which the mitral valve fails to close properly, allowing a backflow of blood. It commonly results from rheumatic heart disease; it may also be a consequence of a heart attack and/or coronary artery disease. It is often asymptomatic, but in advanced cases it can cause shortness of breath and heart failure.	Medications may be prescribed to ease symptoms; in severe cases, valve repair or replacement may be necessary.

Aortic stenosis	Most commonly caused by a deformed valve that narrows over time or, in an elderly person, by deposits of calcium on the valve. As the disorder progresses, it can cause chest pain, fainting, and shortness of breath. Can also occur in young people due to a congenital defect.	Asymptomatic stenosis in adults usually does not require treatment; if symptoms occur, surgical valve replacement is undertaken.
Aortic regurgitation	Tends to be a progressive disorder that may take years to produce symptoms. Possible causes include a congenital defect, rheumatic fever, or infections. Symptoms may include shortness of breath, chest pain, and ankle swelling; untreated, it can lead to an enlarged left ventricle and heart failure.	Symptoms may be eased by taking vasodilator drugs; severe cases, with or without symptoms, call for surgical valve replacement.
Tricuspid regurgitation	This disorder usually accompanies other valve disorders or other heart abnormalities. Isolated trisuspid regurgitation is rare and may be due to a congenital defect. Symptoms may include swelling of the legs and fatigue.	In advanced cases, surgical repair or valve replacement may be needed.
Pulmonary stenosis and regurgitation	These are unusual disorders and are most often congenital in origin. They often accompany other congenital defects.	Surgical treatment or percutaneous valvuloplasty may be needed in a severely narrowed pulmonary valve.

be due to a narrowing, stiffening, or fusing of the valve's leaflets, often caused by a buildup of calcium deposits. Regardless of the cause, the heart is forced to work harder in order to pump blood and meet the body's need for oxygen.

The other major form of heart-valve disease is valvular insufficiency, which is sometimes also called valvular incompetence or regurgitation. The condition develops when a valve fails to close properly and allows a backward flow of a portion of blood that is normally pumped forward to its next destination. Again, the heart is forced to work harder to pump out enough blood. Combined stenosis and insufficiency occurs when the leaflets shrink or stiffen to the degree that the valve is fixed in a partially open position.

Valvular disease most commonly affects the mitral and aortic valves because of the heavy demands placed on them. Over time, valvular disease can lead to heart failure as well as arrhythmias, especially atrial fibrillation. As the heart's workload increases, its muscle compensates by expanding and thickening. For a while the enlarged heart is able to pump enough blood to meet the body's ordinary demands, but eventually the thickened muscle weakens and is unable to pump adequate amounts of blood. This sets the stage for congestive heart failure, a condition in which blood backs up into the lungs and other parts of the body, resulting in fatigue, shortness of breath, swelling (edema), chest pain, and other symptoms.

In the past, rheumatic fever was the leading cause of heart-valve disease; this has changed dramatically thanks to the widespread preventive use of antibiotics. Today, some of the major causes of heart-valve disease are related to aging, such as metabolic changes and calcium deposits. One disorder seen mostly in the elderly is called calcific degeneration. It involves a buildup of calcium deposits, most often on the aortic valve, and also on the ring around the mitral valve, most commonly resulting in aortic stenosis and mitral insufficiency, respectively.

Infective endocarditis is another cause of heart-valve disease. It is an infectious disorder in which bacteria, fungi, or other microorganisms infect the lining of the heart chambers and valves (the endocardium). Unless treated, it can permanently damage the heart's valves and other structures. It is most common among people who already have weakened heart valves, and can often be traced to an untreated infection elsewhere in the body. Drug users who use unsterile techniques (such as sharing hypodermic needles) have an increased risk of developing infective endocarditis.

Coronary artery disease and a heart attack can result in heart-muscle damage that can affect the heart valves or their supporting structures. For example, a heart attack may result in an inability of the mitral valve to close properly, re-sulting in a backflow of blood into the lungs (mitral regurgitation), which can lead to congestive heart failure. Mitral regurgitation can also develop if the left ventricle becomes enlarged, distorting the architecture of the heart and its struc-tures—or if there are excessive and weakened valve structures that degenerate over time (myxomatous degeneration).

Detecting Heart-Valve Disease

A doctor can often detect a defective heart valve simply by listening to the heart through a stethoscope. Blood will flow silently through a healthy heart valve. But if a doctor hears a whooshing noise, commonly called a heart murmur, it may be due to a diseased valve. Stenosis, for example, may be heard as a short, low-pitched murmur; regurgitation may produce a higher-pitched, longer, and softer sound. A clicking sound may point to a valve that fails to close properly; this is especially common in a condition called mitral valve prolapse. An ECG and chest X-ray also provide useful information, especially if valvular disease has re-sulted in an enlarged heart.

The most common diagnostic test, however, is echocardiography (see Chap-ter 6). This painless, noninvasive examination uses high-frequency sound waves to map the heart's internal structures, allowing a doctor to see the shape and mo-tion of the valves. It also enables a doctor to measure the speed and flow of blood through the heart's structures.

The most definitive test may often involve cardiac catheterization and an-giography, especially if heart-valve surgery is being contemplated. This is an in-vasive procedure that involves threading a narrow catheter through the blood vessels and into the heart. A dye is then injected through the catheter and mov-ing X-ray pictures are taken to assess blood flow and the structure of the heart's valves and coronary arteries.

Drug Treatments for Heart-Valve Disease

Treatment of heart-valve disease varies according to the type of disorder. Medica-tions such as vasodilators and diuretics may be prescribed to ease the heart's work-load and to help remove excessive fluid from the body. Mitral regurgitation may be treated, depending on its severity, initially with vasodilators, usually an ACE in-hibitor such as Enalapril; those most likely to benefit are patients who also have high blood pressure. Statins—the drugs used to lower high blood cholesterol—may also be beneficial in patients with aortic stenosis and may prevent further thickening and calcification of the valve.

Blood thinners, or anticoagulants, are prescribed to prevent blood clots, which may form as a consequence of valvular disease complicated by atrial fibrillation. Antiarrhythmic drugs may be used to control an erratic heartbeat, which may be a complication of a defective heart valve. Antibiotics are prescribed prophylactically before dental work, surgery, or other procedures that increase the risk of infection and endocarditis. (See Box 17 on preventive antibiotic therapy.)

Surgical Treatments for Heart-Valve Disease

Several procedures are available to treat advanced or severe heart-valve disease. For example, surgical repair or reconstruction may be considered for severe valvular disease, usually of the mitral or pulmonic or tricuspid valves, that is causing shortness of breath and other symptoms. In severe mitral stenosis, a surgeon

---

Box 17

PREVENTIVE ANTIBIOTIC THERAPY (ENDOCARDITIS PROPHYLAXIS)

People with heart-valve disease have an increased risk of bacterial endocarditis—a serious infection of tissue lining the heart and its valves—when undergoing any dental or surgical procedure in which bacteria or other microorganisms can invade the bloodstream. Be sure that your dentist or any new doctor whom you consult knows you have a heart-valve problem, or if you have been told you have a heart murmur or symptoms of a heart-valve disorder. Endocarditis can be prevented by taking antibiotics before and sometimes after the procedure. For example, the American Heart Association recommends taking three grams of oral amoxicillin (or some other penicillin) an hour before the procedure. In some instances, another dose may be recommended a few hours later. For those unable to take oral medication, the antibiotic can be given by injection.

Persons allergic to penicillin can take erythromycin (typically 800 milligrams) or clindamycin (300 milligrams). Again, depending on the level of risk, a second dose may be prescribed to be taken a few hours after the procedure. Individuals with artificial valves require more extensive regimens.

may physically stretch the leaflets to allow the valve to open more fully. A torn or leaking mitral valve can also be surgically repaired.

If heart-valve disease is causing severe symptoms or is rapidly worsening, or even if there are no symptoms but the heart's size has increased substantially, valve replacement surgery may be recommended. During this operation, a surgeon will remove the diseased valve and replace it with either an artificial (mechanical) valve or one made from animal or human tissue (a biologic valve). There are several types of mechanical valves, which are fashioned from synthetic material, metal, and/or plastics. They tend to last longer—typically twenty years or more—than valves made from living tissue (60 percent of biologic valves have to be replaced after about ten years), but they carry an increased risk of clot formation. To prevent this, patients who have artificial valves usually must take anticoagulant drugs for life.

Goals of Treatment

Treatment is directed at restoring normal valve function and reversing the effects of valve disease on overall heart function.

SUMMING UP

Most of the treatments discussed in this chapter are for life and should never be discontinued without specific guidance from your doctor. Some drugs do produce adverse side effects, but in most instances, the dosages can be adjusted or a suitable, less troubling alternative can be prescribed. Many heart patients take several different medications each day, but this should not be considered a sign that the drugs are not working. As heart disease progresses, additional medications are often needed to treat the changes or prevent serious problems. If you have difficulty remembering to take your medication, talk to your doctor about the possibility of taking combination pills or have your drugs sorted into special medication holders that indicate when you should take each.

Advances in pharmaceutical and surgical treatments for every kind of heart ailment are reasons to feel hopeful about your prospects for an active, happy life after diagnosis. Treatments that would have been unthinkable just a few years ago are rapidly becoming part of mainstream medical practice, giving you and your doctor a growing array of options for improving your condition.

8

Alternative and Complementary Therapies

U ntil about a hundred years ago, doctors and their patients had little choice but to rely largely on folk medicine and herbal remedies to treat illnesses such as cardiovascular disease. This changed radically in the 1900s with the development of the modern pharmaceutical industry and, by the mid-1950s, we had scores of new drugs to treat everything from infections and cancer to diabetes and high blood pressure. Today's pharmacopoeia lists thousands of standardized medications, most of them synthesized from chemical compounds. Most have undergone extensive testing and have been approved by the Food and Drug Administration as safe and effective. Although every drug carries a risk of side effects or adverse reactions, there is no doubt that modern medications have revolutionized medical care.

Nonetheless, alternative remedies—many of them based on ancient folk healing—have reemerged. A study from the Harvard School of Public Health found that, each year, more than 40 percent of Americans resort to some form of alternative medicine. In addition, a growing number of mainstream physicians are incorporating into their practices alternative therapies, usually referred to as complementary or integrative medicine—a movement spearheaded by Dr. Andrew Weil, an Arizona physician who has written a number of best-selling books on natural healing. Popular complementary therapies range from acupuncture, meditation, aromatherapy, yoga, and other facets of traditional Chinese or Eastern medicine, to herbal preparations, high-dose vitamins, homeopathy, and functional foods, among many others.

There is no doubt that alternative or complementary medicine has become a huge business, with Americans spending more than $30 billion a year on these remedies. The array of products is mind-boggling and readily available in supermarkets, pharmacies, and health-food stores, on the Internet, and from numerous other outlets. Many people mistakenly assume that because these products are widely advertised, sold openly, and "natural," they must be safe. But this is not so; serious problems can develop when people self-diagnose and self-treat without consulting a physician. Sampling such products can be especially harmful among people who are also taking prescribed medications to treat some form of cardiovascular disease because many alternative remedies, including nutritional supplements and herbal products, can interact with pharmaceutical drugs (as well as delay the use of known effective treatments).

The experience of Ann, a forty-nine-year-old high school teacher, illustrates the folly of self-treating with popular alternative remedies without medical advice. Ann has high blood pressure and a family history of stroke and heart attacks. She takes three antihypertensive drugs to control her blood pressure, and her doctor has also prescribed a daily baby aspirin—a mild blood thinner—as a preventive measure. When Ann began to experience menopause symptoms, as well as minor joint pain, she started taking high doses of borage oil and ginseng. She added ginkgo biloba pills to improve her memory, and on the suggestion of a friend, also started taking fish oil capsules and 1000 IU of vitamin E a day. To overcome stiffness and joint pain, she often took a couple of over-the-counter anti-inflammatory pills.

Ann became alarmed when she realized that she had a number of unexplained bruises. Her gums were also bleeding a lot, and even a minor cut caused excessive bleeding. When she relayed these symptoms to her doctor, he ordered blood tests, which showed abnormally slow clotting and mild anemia, which further testing traced to a bleeding stomach ulcer. When the doctor asked Ann whether she was taking any supplements or nonprescription medications, he soon learned the source of her bleeding problems. The borage oil, ginkgo, vitamin E, and fish oil supplements, as well as the low-dose aspirin and anti-inflammatory drugs, all have blood-thinning properties, and the combination of so many had suppressed her body's ability to stop bleeding. Fortunately, her blood returned to normal within a few weeks after stopping the supplements. But not all patients are so lucky: Each year, several thousand Americans die because of self-medication with alternative remedies and nonprescription drugs.

All this raises important questions: Is there a place for alternative therapies in your lifelong heart health program? If so, what is it? Again, the answers depend on your individual constants and variables, but some cautions apply to everyone:

1. *Don't automatically assume that if it's natural, it's safe.* Many herbal products carry the same risk of side effects and adverse reactions as their pharmaceutical counterparts, and some are even lethal. For example, ephedra—an herbal product taken to lose weight—caused a number of sudden deaths from cardiac arrhythmias before being banned temporarily in the United States. (Table 16 lists dangerous herbal products.)

2. *Resist the temptation of self-diagnosis and self-treatment with natural remedies.* If you suspect you have a medical problem, consult your doctor. For example, many people who are feeling emotionally down turn to widely publicized and age-old remedies such as St. John's wort or ginkgo biloba and some do, indeed, experience relief. But, as illustrated by Ann's experience, they can interact with each other and with prescribed medications. In addition, true clinical depression should be diagnosed and treated by a mental health professional.

3. *Let your doctor know everything you're taking and trying, including vitamins, minerals, and herbal products.* Many of these reduce or increase the effectiveness of prescribed drugs. For example, large amounts of calcium and high-fiber supplements can interfere with the absorption of some antibiotics and other drugs. Hawthorne, a popular herbal remedy for heart disease, can increase the effect of antihypertensive drugs, and result in dizziness and other symptoms of low blood pressure.

4. *Never stop taking a prescribed medication in order to take an alternative therapy reputed to have the same effect.* For example, some herbal and nutraceutical products are promoted as effective in reducing cholesterol or lowering high blood pressure. Although these claims may have some validity, most herbal or so-called natural remedies have not been subjected to scientific testing, and their content is not standardized, so dosages can vary widely. Always check with your doctor before making any change in your treatment program.

Having raised a number of red flags, we turn to the more positive side of alternative or complementary medicine. When approached with common sense and in consultation with a knowledgeable health professional, a number of these practices can be incorporated safely into your total regimen. Indeed, some may be

TABLE 16

HERBAL PRODUCTS DANGEROUS TO THE CARDIOVASCULAR SYSTEM

Plant source	Folk uses	Dangers
Blue cohosh (*Caulophyllum thalictroides*; should not be confused with black cohosh, or *Cimicifuga racemosa*)	Menstrual irregularities, muscle spasms	Can cause serious heart damage and raise blood pressure. Seeds are poisonous and berries and roots can damage cells.
Ephedra (*Ephedra sinica*) or ma huang (once banned but again sold in the United States)	Weight loss, asthma, airway constriction	Can raise blood pressure, speed the heartbeat, and lead to a heart attack, stroke, or sudden death.
Dong quai (*Angelica polymorphia, A. sinesis,* and *A. acutiloba*)	General tonic, female ginseng	Contains natural coumarine compounds that can cause serious bleeding problems.
Foxglove (*Digitalis purpurea* and others)	Historically, used to treat edema (dropsy) and advanced heart disease; digitalis is now synthesized chemically so the dosage can be carefully controlled.	Digitalis glycosides can be highly toxic and even a small overdose can cause cardiac arrhythmias, dizziness, confusion, convulsions, visual side effects, and even death.
Licorice (*Glycyrrhiza glabra*)	Relieve cold symptoms, heartburn, PMS	Can raise blood pressure and promote fluid retention.
Lobelia (*Lobelia inflata*)	Expectorant, alleviate symptoms of nicotine withdrawal	Palpitations, dizziness, vomiting, and other intestinal symptoms; taken in a large dose, it can result in a drop in blood pressure, shock, coma, and death.
Pennyroyal (*Hedeoma pulegioides*)	Cold and flu symptoms; induce abortion	Palpitation, high blood pressure, liver damage, shock, and possible death.
Pokeweed (*Phytolacca americana*)	General "cleansing" tonic; skin ulcers, hemorrhoids, infection	Drop in blood pressure, confusion, convulsions, vomiting, and impaired breathing.
Yohimbe (*Pausinystalia yohimbe*)	Male and female aphrodisiac; male impotence	Overdose can cause panic, tremors, rise in blood pressure; higher doses can cause drop in blood pressure, weakness, and even paralysis.

preferable to pharmaceutical products or other interventions. For example, relaxation therapies—meditation, yoga and other movement modalities, therapeutic massage, and aromatherapy—can counter the harmful effects of daily stress.

NUTRACEUTICALS AND FUNCTIONAL FOODS

In the last few years, a growing number of physicians and other health professionals have adopted a more positive approach to nutraceuticals: substances derived from plants or other organic products, but which are taken in amounts much higher than you can get from an ordinary diet. For example, very high doses of folic acid—one of the B-complex vitamins—is the mainstream treatment for elevated homocysteine, an amino acid (protein) that may raise the risk of a heart attack when larger than normal amounts circulate in the blood. Still, you should consult your doctor or a qualified nutritionist before taking any high-dose vitamin or mineral. Some, such as vitamins A and D and iron, can be toxic when taken in large amounts, and others, such as calcium, can interfere with the metabolism of prescribed medications.

So-called functional foods have gained increasing popularity in recent years, thanks largely to extensive advertising and articles in the popular press. These include Benecol, a canola-based margarine that is promoted to lower cholesterol; coenzyme Q_{10}, which is said to improve circulation and reduce the risk of blood clots; the flavonoids in green tea, soy beans, red wine, and berries, which may lower the risk of a heart attack; and oat bran, which may lower cholesterol and improve blood sugar control. These and a number of other potential functional foods, including chocolate, are undergoing scientific studies, and some preliminary results appear promising (see Box 18). But caution is still needed, because dosages usually are not standardized and they are not subjected to the same quality control standards as FDA-approved products. (Table 17 lists a selection of nutraceuticals and functional foods that may be useful in treating or preventing cardiovascular disorders.)

HERBAL PRODUCTS

Herbs are yet another source of increasingly popular alternative therapies. Worldwide, these substances are by far the most used medicines, and even in developed countries like the United States, many pharmaceutical drugs are based on plant products. Many researchers believe that as yet undiscovered botanicals may provide cures for some of our most lethal diseases, and toward this end,

Box 18

HOW BITTERSWEET IT IS

Chocolate—long heralded as the food of the gods and a token of love—is fast emerging as a functional food that is said to treat or prevent cardiovascular disease, memory loss, depression, chronic fatigue, and a host of other ailments. Is this just another food fad? Maybe, but there is mounting scientific evidence that chocolate may indeed have health benefits.

Cocoa beans are rich in flavonoids, naturally occurring antioxidant compounds found in many foods and beverages, including red wine, tea, and a variety of brightly colored fruits, berries, and vegetables. Ongoing studies indicate that cocoa flavonoids (flavonols) may lower blood pressure by widening or relaxing small blood vessels. These flavonols, as well as the heart-healthy fats in cocoa butter, help prevent the buildup of fatty deposits in the arteries. They appear to increase blood flow to the brain, which may improve memory. Flavonols and other flavonoids reduce blood clot formation by inhibiting platelet clumping. The caffeine in cocoa promotes mental alertness; cocoa also contains chemicals that elevate mood and perhaps dull pain by increasing the brain's production of endorphins.

A group at Harvard Medical School, led by Dr. Norman K. Hollenberg, have studied residents of Kuna, an island off Panama, who drink about five cups of cocoa a day and also consume cocoa in many foods. High blood pressure is virtually unknown among these people, but their risk of hypertension and heart disease rises when they leave the island and forgo their cocoa-rich diet.

A few words of caution, however, before you reach for a chocolate bar. Processing cocoa beans (roasting, fermentation, alkalizing) into palatable chocolate destroys large amounts of its flavonols. The addition of sugar adds empty calories, promotes weight gain, and raises blood sugar (glucose). So by the time cocoa is transformed into candy, it's hardly a health food. The most benefits are derived from dark unsweetened chocolate, or bittersweet made with a sugar substitute. Many people find this type of chocolate too bitter or pungent. Chocolate manufacturers are looking for ways of retaining flavonols and overcoming the natural bitterness of cocoa. In the meantime, it's comforting to know that you needn't feel guilty about occasionally indulging in a few ounces of dark chocolate. Look for brands that are at least 70 percent cocoa and low in added sugar.

TABLE 17

SOME NUTRACEUTICALS, FUNCTIONAL FOODS, AND HERBAL PRODUCTS
PROMOTED FOR HEART HEALTH

Product	Available as	Purported Benefits
Benecol	Margarine	May lower total cholesterol and raise beneficial LDL cholesterol.
Beta glucans	Mushroom extracts, baker's yeast, beta 1,3/1,6 glucan (such as Norwegian Beta 1,3/1,6 Glucan)	May lower cholesterol.
Cinnamon (*Connamomum zeylanicum/cassia*)	Bark or ground spice	May increase insulin uptake in persons with type II diabetes.
Coenzyme Q_{10} or CoQ	Tablets, pills, capsules	May ease symptoms of heart failure (shortness of breath, edema, difficulty sleeping); may also slow progression of degenerative nerve disease.
Essential fatty acids (linoleic, alpha-linolenic acid, omega 3 and 6 fatty acids)	Abundant in salmon and other cold-water fish; sold as fish oil gel caps and liquid supplements	May lower risk of heart attacks and strokes; lowers blood levels of cholesterol and triglycerides; may aid in treatment of arthritis and depression.
Flavonoids	Green tea, soybeans, red wines, dark chocolate, many fruits and vegetables; also available as supplements and soy protein	May reduce risk of a heart attack.
Flax (*Linum usitatissimum*)	Ground seeds, gel caps of flax oil	May lower blood cholesterol; helps prevent constipation; may ease arthritis inflammation and pain.
Garlic (*Allium sativum*)	Fresh herb, powder, or pill supplements	May help lower blood pressure and blood cholesterol; mild blood thinner that can cause platelet dysfunction; may enhance immunity.

Product	Available as	Purported Benefits
Ginkgo (*Ginkgo biloba*)	Standardized extract	May improve circulation by widening peripheral blood vessels; may lower blood pressure and reduce clotting risk.
Glucomannan (*Konjac* or *Konjac mannan*)	High-fiber powder	May lower blood cholesterol; enhances blood sugar control; aids in weight loss by promoting feeling of fullness.
Guggul (*Commiphora mukul*)	Standardized guggulsterone extract	Contains gugulipid, which may lower blood cholesterol.
Hawthorne (*Crataegus species*)	Elixirs, extracts, infusion, capsules, tinctures, and teas from dried leaves	Contains flavonoids and other compounds that widen blood vessels; may lower blood pressure and reduce swelling in heart failure.
L-arginine	Amino acid found in meat and high-protein foods; as a supplement, sold as capsules and pills	May improve circulation in people with intermittent claudication (leg pain during exercise due to reduced blood flow).
Lecithin	Fatty compound found in all body cells; dietary sources include egg yolks and soybeans, meat, especially organ meats; supplements include pills, capsules, softgels, powders, and liquid	May enhance effectiveness of clofibrate, a cholesterol lowering drug; may also protect intestinal tract against damage from aspirin and other anti-inflammatory drugs.
Oat bran	Oatmeal and other cereals made from whole oats; oat bran powder and pills	May lower blood cholesterol, improve blood sugar control.
Psyllium seed (*Plantago psyllium*)	Metamucil and other psyllium laxatives, powders, pills, and capsules	May lower harmful LDL cholesterol; aids in weight control by promoting feeling of fullness.
Red rice yeast (*Monascus purpureus*)	Cholestin capsules	Contains a chemical similar to that found in statin drugs; may lower blood cholesterol and triglycerides and raise levels of beneficial HDL cholesterol.

they are searching rain forests and other remaining natural environments for potential medicines.

Very few of the hundreds of herbal medicines available today have been subjected to scientific testing for safety and effectiveness. The amounts of active ingredients in a given product vary greatly from one manufacturer to another, and even from batch to batch. In contrast, pharmaceutical products are synthesized from chemical compounds and dosages can be controlled with great precision. Practitioners and advocates of herbal medicine contend that their substances, many of which have been used for centuries, have stood the test of time and are generally safer than pharmaceuticals—but this assertion is open to debate. Many herbal products are harmless and may or may not be effective, while others are dangerous and should not be used or should be approached with great caution. As a general rule, do not take any medicine—herbal, prescription, or over-the-counter—without first consulting an expert, preferably your doctor or a health professional (for example, pharmacist, registered dietitian, or other licensed practitioner).

Common Forms of Herbal Remedies

Tinctures are extracts of dried or fresh plants that are preserved in alcohol. They are generally very concentrated, and should be diluted before consuming. Freeze-dried extracts, by contrast, are prepared by flash freezing to evaporate the fluid from the plant. Alternatively, the active ingredients may be extracted with chemicals and then freeze dried to remove the chemical solvents. Freeze-dried extracts are packaged in capsules; dosages may or may not be standardized depending on the product and manufacturer.

In addition, loose herbs may be available in fresh or dried forms, and many are sold in bulk to be brewed into teas. The effective ingredients often deteriorate rapidly due to exposure to light, air, and moisture. Fermenting—a process used in preparing many dried teas—helps preserve some of the beneficial ingredients, such as flavonoids. Harmful ingredients, however, such as pesticides and other environmental contaminants, may also persist and even be concentrated by the drying process. To guard against the danger of consuming such contaminants, look for products from reputable manufacturers and those that are organically grown.

If you are looking for topical (external) herbal preparations, you will find many poultices, salves, ointments, and lotions from which to choose. Aloe vera is a common example of an herbal product that is applied topically to the skin.

Some herbal products, such as comfrey, that are dangerous when ingested, may be used safely as a topical preparation.

Herbal Aphrodisiacs

A number of herbal products are promoted as natural sex enhancers or aphrodisiacs. Heart patients are tempted to turn to these aids for a number of reasons. For example, many also have diabetes—a disease that often causes sexual dysfunction. Some of the medications used to treat high blood pressure and other cardiovascular disorders, too, can interfere with sexual function. Depression, a disorder that commonly develops after a heart attack, stroke, or heart surgery, is still another source of sexual problems.

Scores of so-called natural sex boosters are widely available on the internet, in vitamin and health food stores, even supermarkets and pharmacies. These include ginseng root, horny goat weed (*Epimedium sagittatum* or yin yang huo), damiana (*Turnera diffusa*), yohimbine, and many others. While some of these are seemingly harmless and may or may not be of any real benefit, others, such as yohimbine, are very toxic substances that should never be used. Horny goat weed, an herb that grows in Asia and Mediterranean countries, has long been used as a sex enhancer in China but has been marketed for only a few years in the United States. Despite claims of safety, it should be avoided or used with great caution by heart patients because it may provoke cardiac arrhythmias. Many herbal products contain ingredients that can raise blood pressure or interact with heart medications. Some also contain hormones that can be harmful. There are much safer alternatives to these products. If you are experiencing a sexual problem, discuss it with your doctor. A prescription drug such as sildenafil (Viagra), varenafil (Levitra), or tadalafil (Cialis) may be appropriate; if not, there are a number of other approaches that can be tried. A word of warning, however: none of these drugs should ever be used by a patient who is also taking nitroglycerin or any nitroglycerine preparation or derivative such as isosorbide mononitrate to control chest pains and other cardiac symptoms. The combination has been known to provoke a marked fall in blood pressure, or shock, which can prove fatal.

SUMMING UP

Millions of Americans, including heart patients, routinely turn to herbal medicine, nutraceuticals, and other forms of complementary medicine. Although some of these products are harmless or even beneficial, others are potentially dangerous. Always check with your doctor or other health professional before resorting to alternative remedies, especially if you are also taking prescribed medications: even if the health aids are touted as "natural" or "safe," they can cause serious and harmful side effects or interactions.

PART

III

Populations
with
Special
Concerns

Throughout this book, we've emphasized the importance of creating a lifelong heart-care program that is suited to your individual needs. In developing this personalized approach, you may benefit from learning about groups that require special strategies for improving heart health. For example, advancing age is an important consideration, and treatment of heart disease in the elderly may be quite different from that in a young person. Not only is heart disease itself more severe among the elderly, but its long-term treatment is likely to be affected by changing physiology and by coexisting diseases that become increasingly common as we age.

It is also becoming clear that gender plays a role in the treatment and prevention of heart disease, a condition that can have different symptoms and characteristics in women than in men. By increasing the number of women in clinical studies, we are learning that what works well for a male patient may not be the best choice for his female counterpart. Pregnancy, too, affects the cardiovascular system and sometimes results in serious, even life-threatening problems. Eating disorders, which are increasingly common among young women, can damage the heart as well.

Patients' ethnic, racial, and cultural backgrounds also pose special issues in diagnosing and treating heart disease. At one time it was assumed that as minority groups assimilated into the majority population, their risks and disease profiles would mirror those of other Americans. But this is not the case, and race and ethnic or cultural heritage must be considered when developing an effective treatment and preventive program for African Americans, Hispanics, Native Americans, and other minority populations.

Although relatively rare, heart disease in young athletes frequently garners headlines and is a source of concern not only for the young people involved, but also for parents and coaches. Improved treatment of congenital heart disease has enabled an increasing number of babies born with these defects to reach adulthood. Treating these patients presents special challenges, often requiring care supervised by specialists. Finally, heart patients sometimes face special risks when traveling, especially when visiting high altitudes. Still, with advance planning and common sense, most heart patients can now enjoy travel to most places. The following chapters provide a brief overview of special challenges faced by these populations.

9

Heart Care for Women

Cardiovascular disease is by far the leading cause of death of American women, accounting for more than 493,000 deaths a year compared to about 433,000 fatalities among men. Yet all too often, cardiovascular disease goes undiagnosed or undertreated in this population group. Why? Doctors must share part of the blame because they often overlook the warning signs or downplay risk factors in their female patients, which can result in delaying treatment until the disease reaches an advanced stage. Furthermore, the biology of cardiovascular disease and its symptoms are often different in women than men.

Women themselves are also, at least in part, responsible for such delays. Ask any woman to name the disease that's most likely to cause her death, and chances are she will immediately reply "breast cancer," even though it accounts for about forty thousand deaths a year—only a fraction of the toll from cardiovascular disease. Ask the same woman to name her top health concern about her husband and she's likely to say a heart attack. She's conscientious about having regular mammograms and breast and gynecology checkups for herself, and in her role of family caregiver, she is likely to make sure that her husband has his cholesterol and blood pressure checked. While all this is prudent, it overlooks what should be the woman's top health concern—namely, the state of her own heart health. Let's take a brief look at a few startling facts:

♥ One in every eight or nine women aged forty-five to sixty-four has some form of cardiovascular disease. After age sixty-five, the number jumps to one in three.

♥ About half of all fatal heart attacks occur in women, but a woman who has a heart attack has a twofold risk of dying within the first two weeks, compared to her male counterpart. This is especially true for women under the age of forty-five.

♥ High blood pressure—a major risk factor for heart attack and stroke—is more prevalent among women than men, and the likelihood of developing it rises sharply with age.

♥ Hormonal and other changes occurring during pregnancy can lead to high blood pressure, which should be carefully monitored. Although pregnancy-related high blood pressure usually returns to normal following childbirth, these women have an increased risk of becoming hypertensive in their later years.

♥ Obesity and diabetes are more common among women than men and, according to the American Heart Association, these risk factors are about twice as dangerous for women—especially African American women—as for men. This fact takes on additional significance when you consider that more than a third of American women are obese, and their numbers are increasing each year.

♥ Tobacco use clearly increases risk of premature death in both sexes, but in women it appears to carry special cardiovascular risks. Nicotine is more addictive in women than men, making it more difficult for women to quit. Women who smoke are six to nine times more likely to suffer a heart attack compared to nonsmokers. The combined use of oral contraceptives and cigarette smoking greatly increases the risk of developing blood clots that can lead to a stroke or heart attack. Tobacco erases the presumed protective effect of estrogen among premenopausal women, and at any age it promotes a rise in the harmful LDL cholesterol and accelerates the buildup of fatty deposits in the arteries (atherosclerosis).

♥ Women, especially as they age, tend to be more sedentary than men, and are less likely to adopt a regular exercise and fitness regimen.

HORMONE REPLACEMENT THERAPY

Until menopause, women enjoy a statistical edge over their male counterparts when it comes to cardiovascular disease. This advantage begins to decline with menopause, and by age sixty-five, the number of women with some form of cardiovascular disease is about equal to that of men. Estrogen—the main female sex hormone—has long been credited with protecting the cardiovascular system, and it undoubtedly plays a role. For example, young women tend to have a more favorable ratio of HDL (beneficial) to LDL (harmful) cholesterol—a balance that changes markedly after menopause. In addition, women tend to accumulate more abdominal fat after menopause, as well as have an accelerated rate of atherosclerosis and an increased risk of diabetes. As noted, hypertension also becomes more prevalent after menopause.

These observations of the presumed protective effects of estrogen led to a widespread assumption that hormone replacement therapy (HRT) after menopause would continue the protective effect of estrogen. Although the data are mixed, ongoing studies indicate that this is not the case; in fact, postmenopausal estrogen replacement appears to increase the risk of a stroke and heart attack as well as certain cancers while offering little or no protection against heart disease. The Women's Health Initiative Study, an ongoing research project involving thousands of women, found that for every ten thousand women taking HRT, thirty-seven would suffer heart attacks in the course of a year, seven more than among women not taking the hormones. These findings are contrary to a 1989 report from the Nurses' Health Study, which has followed more than 48,000 postmenopausal women. This study, first reported in 1989, found that women on HRT had fewer heart attacks than those not taking hormones. The reasons for the discrepancies are unclear, but explanations are being sought through further research. At present, HRT may be needed to treat symptoms of estrogen withdrawal (night sweats, hot flashes, mood swings, and others); it may also protect bones against osteoporosis (although there are a number of effective estrogen alternatives for this). But any potential benefit clearly must be weighed against the possible risk. In any event, HRT should not be taken to prevent cardiovascular disease. When HRT is prescribed, it should be given in the lowest effective dosage needed to control symptoms, and the woman should be gradually taken off of it as soon as possible.

PSYCHOLOGICAL AND SOCIAL ISSUES

Psychological and social issues also appear to work against women. Older women are more likely to live alone than men, meaning they may lack the social support that is so important in altering risk factors and adopting an effective long-term program. Even women who live with others are often cast in a caregiver role, leading them to ignore or neglect their own needs. Women who work outside the home typically have at least two jobs—their outside employment as well as responsibility for child-care and household chores, a combination that often leads to high levels of stress. Women are also more likely to suffer from depression, which may also increase cardiovascular risk or result in a woman's tendency to deny heart symptoms or neglect treatment.

DIAGNOSIS AND TREATMENT

For both men and women, the best approach to heart disease is to prevent its onset, and if chest pains, shortness of breath, and other symptoms occur, to seek immediate medical attention. Women lag behind men in cardiovascular screening. A woman's regular health checkup should include cholesterol screening and testing of blood glucose levels. She should also have a resting ECG every five to ten years starting at age twenty or twenty-five. Certain stages of the menstrual cycle can result in transient abnormalities, both at rest and during exercise. These can mimic changes characteristic of coronary artery disease. Thus, a woman should let her doctor know the date of her last period when undergoing an ECG or stress test.

Women who have two or more cardiovascular risk factors or symptoms suggesting possible heart disease may be advised to also undergo an exercise stress test with imaging. A routine exercise ECG is more likely to produce false positive results in women than men. This discrepancy can be reduced by stress echocardiography or radionuclide imaging, which tend to improve diagnostic accuracy.

Unfortunately, when a woman is diagnosed as having coronary artery disease or another cardiovascular problem, the disorder has often progressed to an advanced stage. Even when a woman sees a doctor because of chest pains, shortness of breath, and other symptoms of coronary artery disease, her heart problem may go undiagnosed. There are a number of reasons for this oversight. For example, atypical angina—chest pains that occur during rest or during mental stress—or pain that seems to arise in the back or stomach may be misdiagnosed as anxiety or other medical problems. In addition, men with atypical angina are much more likely than women to be referred for coronary angiography—the gold standard diagnostic test for coronary artery disease. This is one area in which women should be more assertive; if you suspect you have a heart problem, don't be put off with assurances that "it's probably just stress or overwork," or "you're too young to have heart disease." If necessary, ask for a referral to a cardiologist who is experienced in treating women as well as men. But it's important to remember that not every chest pain or other potential heart-related symptom originates in the cardiovascular system; prudence and common sense can foster a proper balance between too little and too much caution. Also, resist the temptation of going from doctor to doctor until you hear what you want to hear; second and even third opinions can be valuable, but there should be a sound reason for seeking them.

DIFFERENCES IN TREATMENT

Women suffering a heart attack often experience different symptoms than men do. When pain occurs, it may be centered more in the neck, jaw, back, or abdomen than in the chest itself, and the profuse sweating that typically accompanies a heart attack in a man is less likely to occur. In addition, "silent" or painless heart attacks are more common among older women than among men.

Although both men and women having a heart attack typically wait several hours before seeking medical help, women often delay even longer. Thus by the time they arrive at the hospital, it may be too late for treatment with clot-dissolving drugs. When such medications are given early in the course of a heart attack, however, they are just as effective in minimizing heart damage in women as in men.

Heretofore, doctors thought women were less likely than men to benefit from angioplasty and stents to open clogged arteries. Studies done during the past few years, however, indicate that these aggressive treatments are equally effective in both men and women (especially if drug-eluting stents—devices that are impregnated with drugs that prevent growth of tissue in the blood vessel walls—are used). In contrast, coronary artery bypass surgery in certain instances may be less likely to benefit women, because women often have smaller coronary arteries than men.

Following a heart attack, men are more likely than women to undergo intensive cardiac rehabilitation, perhaps because women tend to be older, frailer, and have coexisting diseases that make rehabilitation more difficult. Still, there is no doubt that even these older, sicker women can benefit from rehab and adoption of a long-term program that includes behavior modification—namely, increased physical activity, a more healthful diet, and smoking cessation.

Low-Dose Aspirin for Women

Numerous studies show that low-dose aspirin—for example, one baby aspirin or half of a regular tablet—can help prevent heart attacks in men. But this does not appear to hold true for women, at least those under the age of sixty-five. Results of a ten-year study that followed forty thousand women over the age of forty-five showed no significant protective effect against heart attacks, although there was some protection against strokes caused by blood clots. In contrast, men who took a preventive low-dose aspirin enjoyed a 44 percent reduction in heart-attack risk, but little or no protection against a stroke. The reason for these differences is unclear, but some attribute it to the fact that women have smaller coronary arteries than men and thus are more susceptible to blockage of a blood clot even if taking aspirin. Because even low-dose aspirin increases the risk of bleeding and stomach problems, these factors should be weighed carefully before a woman starts aspirin therapy. In any event, she should not do so without first consulting her doctor.

PREGNANCY-RELATED HEART PROBLEMS

Just a few decades ago, women with almost any type of heart disease were discouraged from attempting pregnancy, and with good reason. In this era before antibiotics, rheumatic fever was a common affliction that left many people with severely damaged heart valves. Today, rheumatic fever is almost unknown in developed countries, and other forms of cardiovascular disease that once rendered pregnancy life-threatening often can now be treated. Consequently, a woman with heart disease can now often attempt pregnancy with reduced fear for her life or the life of her baby. Even so, 1 to 4 percent of all pregnancies in the United States are complicated by cardiovascular disorders (not including preexisting heart conditions such as congenital defects or valvular disease). Such pregnancies are considered high-risk and the woman must be carefully monitored at all stages.

Even under normal circumstances, pregnancy puts a strain on the entire cardiovascular system. For example, during a normal pregnancy a woman's blood volume increases by 40 to 50 percent, forcing the heart to beat faster and harder to circulate the extra blood. Without extra iron to form hemoglobin—the pigment that carries oxygen in the blood—a woman is at high risk of developing pregnancy-related anemia. This can lead to fatigue, shortness of breath, and other symptoms.

Although blood pressure normally falls somewhat during a normal pregnancy, about 20 percent of pregnancies are complicated by hypertension, defined as consistent blood pressure readings of 140/90 or higher. This high blood pressure may be preexisting, in which case it should be carefully monitored and treated before and throughout the pregnancy. But some women who have normal blood pressure also experience an increase; this is referred to as gestational hypertension and is most common during the last trimester or at the time of delivery. It may persist for several weeks after delivery, and follow-up studies indicate that these women have an increased risk of developing chronic hypertension later in life.

Increased blood pressure is also a component of preeclampsia, a complication that develops in 3 to 8 percent of pregnancies in the United States. The typical symptoms include a rise in blood pressure, swelling (edema), and protein in the urine. These symptoms may come on gradually during the third trimester or develop abruptly at the time of delivery. In any event, the condition should be monitored even though it usually resolves itself after delivery. A much more serious complication is eclampsia, a condition in which a woman with preeclampsia develops seizures and other serious, even life-threatening symptoms. In such cases, the baby is delivered immediately and the woman undergoes intensive treatment to control blood pressure, seizures, and other complications.

Another pregnancy-related heart disorder—peripartum cardiomyopathy or PPCM—is relatively rare, occurring in one of every three to four thousand births in the United States. The condition typically develops in the later stages of pregnancy and as late as five months after delivery. The symptoms—fatigue, shortness of breath, possible chest pain, abdominal discomfort and distension, and water retention in the lungs and other parts of the body—are often attributed to changes that occur toward the end of pregnancy. A cardiovascular exam and echocardiogram can establish the diagnosis, and treatment generally is similar to that of other heart-muscle disorders (or "cardiomyopathies"; see Chapter 7). Fifty to 60 percent of women with PPCM recover completely within six months, but others may continue to decline and will require long-term treatment. After recovery, there is an increased risk for PPCM in subsequent pregnancies. Patients who do not recover should not undergo additional pregnancies.

Another unusual complication of pregnancy involves a spontaneous dissection of the coronary artery. This can result in peripartum angina or heart attack.

Complications of Pregnancy in Women with Preexisting Heart Disease

Preexisting heart conditions can be classified according to the degree of threat they pose to the mother or her fetus. Of low risk are the following disorders:

💜 *Mitral valve prolapse.* This condition, in which the leaflets that make up the mitral valve are larger than normal, rarely poses a problem in pregnancy.

💜 *Mitral regurgitation.* This condition is characterized by a failure of the mitral valve to close properly, allowing a backflow of blood. It is generally well tolerated during pregnancy, although women with severe mitral regurgitation are advised to undergo surgical repair before attempting to have a baby.

💜 *Aortic regurgitation.* With mild forms of this condition, in which the aortic valve fails to close properly, pregnancy is generally well tolerated. But in severe aortic regurgitation, surgical repair or valve replacement should be carried out before conception.

💜 *Premature ventricular and/or atrial beats.* These mild cardiac arrhythmias usually do not pose a problem during pregnancy, but the more severe (and rare) conditions of atrial fibrillation and atrial flutter may require treatment, with either medication or electrical cardioversion—a procedure to restore a normal heartbeat.

Conditions that pose a moderate risk for pregnant women include:

💜 *Mitral stenosis.* This condition, characterized by a narrowing or stiffening of the mitral valve, can cause serious complications during the third trimester or during labor and delivery. Women with mild mitral stenosis should be monitored carefully during pregnancy, and treated if the condition worsens.

💜 *Aortic stenosis.* In this condition, the aortic valve is narrowed or stiffened. Like mitral stenosis it requires careful monitoring during pregnancy. Severe aortic stenosis should be corrected before conception.

Pregnancy should not be attempted by women with these high-risk preexisting conditions:

💜 *Primary pulmonary hypertension (PPH).* This condition involves abnormally high blood pressure in the arteries that supply the lungs.

💜 *Severe congenital heart defects.* These defects include those that result in cyanosis, a bluish tinge of the skin caused by insufficient oxygenation, as well as those that involve significant pulmonary hypertension, Marfan syndrome, or a dilated aortic root. Generally, less severe but significant defects that are amenable to surgery should be operated on prior to pregnancy (see Chapter 13).

EATING DISORDERS AND THE HEART

An estimated 8 million Americans suffer from serious eating disorders; of these, the overwhelming majority—about 7 million—are girls and young women. Recent studies indicate that 20 to 25 percent of college-age women engage in binging and purging—hallmarks of bulimia. Overall, however, about 4 to 5 percent of American women will, at some point in their lives, be bulimic or engage in binge eating and purging. A smaller number, an estimated 1 to 3.7 percent of all females, will suffer from anorexia nervosa, a serious eating disorder characterized by self-starvation and a grossly distorted body image.

Types of Eating Disorders

It is sometimes difficult to distinguish between eating disorders, fad diets, and borderline adolescent behavior. In general, however, anorexia nervosa is characterized by serious weight loss achieved by self-starvation, induced vomiting, abuse of laxatives or diuretics, and perhaps compulsive exercise. Bulimia nervosa, a related disorder, features recurrent episodes of compulsive binge eating, usually followed by purging through self-induced vomiting, excessive exercise, and fasting. (Surprisingly, the person's weight may be normal.) Binge eating disorders involve recurrent (two or more times a week) episodes of compulsive overeating, but without the purging of anorexia nervosa and bulimia nervosa. The patient's weight may range from normal to obese.

These eating disorders have a very high mortality rate; without treatment, as many as 20 percent of patients die. With treatment, about 60 percent recover and the death rate falls to 2 to 3 percent. But even with treatment, about 20 percent recover only partially and another 20 percent do not improve. The causes of eating disorders are not fully understood, but likely include psychological problems, social and family issues, and hormonal changes and other physical factors. The consequences are more clear-cut, however, especially in the ways that these disorders affect the heart. In fact, heart disease is the most common cause of death among people with eating disorders, especially anorexia nervosa. Eating disorders have many effects on the cardiovascular system. For example, anorexia can cause a slow heartbeat (bradycardia), which can result in dizziness, fatigue, and fainting. The dehydration and starvation that occur in anorexia also can result in an imbalance in electrolytes, especially calcium and potassium. These minerals are essential in maintaining a normal heartbeat; an imbalance can result in serious cardiac arrhythmias and even cardiac arrest.

The dehydration associated with anorexia and frequent purging can also reduce blood volume, resulting in low blood pressure and poor circulation. In contrast to anorexia nervosa, bulimia may result in high blood pressure. For all eating disorders, the lack of adequate nutrition can result in anemia and other blood disorders.

During starvation, the body starts to break down and use its own lean tissue, including the heart muscle. This can result in a reduced heart size and set the stage for cardiac arrest. In addition, bulimia and binge eating disorders often result in elevated cholesterol, especially the harmful LDL cholesterol, thus increasing the risk of coronary artery disease.

Of course, eating disorders have detrimental effects on other body systems, resulting in hormonal changes, menstrual and fertility problems, digestive disorders, nerve damage, bone loss, and an increased risk of depression and other psychological disorders. Experts agree that the best approach entails early recognition, diagnosis, and intensive treatment, which may involve the entire family.

SUMMING UP

Cardiovascular disease is by far the leading cause of death among American women, yet many go undiagnosed and untreated until a heart attack, stroke, or other major cardiac event occurs. Heart disease in women often causes symptoms that are different from those experienced by men; women may also require different approaches to treatment. Even so, increased awareness of the danger and early preventive measures can keep more women from falling victim to heart disease.

10

Heart Disease in the Elderly

Thanks to modern medicine, along with improved nutrition and sanitation, people in developed countries are living longer, healthier lives. Indeed, the elderly make up the fastest growing segment of the American population, with more than 35 million Americans over the age of sixty-five and some 10 million over age eighty. By 2030, more than 70 million Americans will fall into the over-sixty-five set. But even though today's elderly are healthier than in past generations, there's no escaping the fact that as we age, we are increasingly vulnerable to a host of ailments, including cardiovascular disease.

HOW OLD IS OLD?

Bob Hope often quipped that an elderly person was anyone ten years your senior. Joking aside, the definition of elderly has changed in recent decades. Not long ago, old age was thought to begin at age fifty or fifty-five. Today, the World Health Organization designates sixty as elderly and the United States generally settles on sixty-five. But just what constitutes elderly varies greatly from one person to another. Many people in their late sixties and seventies enjoy the vigor and health more typical of middle age; in contrast, there are people in their fifties who are afflicted with problems associated with the aged, making them feel, act, and look like they are much older than they are. Whatever your actual age, physiology trumps chronology.

In medical practice, treatment decisions cannot be based on age alone, but must also take into consideration your overall health and physical fitness, coexisting diseases, and mental attitude and acuity. Today's increased emphasis on healthful lifestyles and improved medical care mean that increasing numbers of elderly persons are enjoying good health, and when heart disease does develop, they usually can undergo even aggressive treatment. John, the eighty-five-year-old retiree introduced earlier, is a case in point. John winters in Florida and spends the spring and summer months in New England. Although he has long-standing hypertension and moderately elevated blood cholesterol levels, he controls both with medication. He has always been active, playing golf several times a week and enjoying long walks with his wife and dog. He first started experiencing chest pains when climbing stairs or walking at a brisk pace. At first, he attributed the symptoms to "getting old," but at the urging of his daughter, he consulted his doctor. Tests revealed that John had severe coronary artery disease, making him a prime candidate for a heart attack.

John asked his doctor whether his advanced age precluded surgery or other aggressive treatment. The doctor assured John that he was not too old, and given the state and safety of modern heart surgery, he was a good candidate for bypass surgery. After some hesitation, John elected to undergo the surgery, which was successful. In just a few months, he was back on the golf course and going about his normal routine free of chest pain.

John's story illustrates that age is not a barrier to treating even severe heart disease. While the risk of surgery is moderately increased in those beyond eighty, in general, a patient's physiologic and clinical state is much more important than absolute age in the decision whether to operate. In the United States, for example, one-forth of all angioplasty procedures and bypass operations are performed in patients seventy-five or older. But it's also important to recognize some of the effects of aging on cardiac function. Here are a few generalizations:

- ♥ Although the human heart is designed to last a lifetime, subtle changes do occur with advancing age. For example, the older heart may lose some of its responsiveness to adrenaline, and it may not be able to beat as fast or strongly during exercise. These changes may not be noticeable in a person who has retained a good level of cardiovascular fitness, in contrast to those who are sedentary and may already have some degree of coronary artery disease.
- ♥ The prevalence of heart disease increases markedly with advancing age. Cardiovascular disorders make up the most common diagnoses and cause of death among people over age sixty-five, and the prevalence increases

with age. For example, cardiovascular disease accounts for 60 percent of deaths among people over the age of seventy-five. Autopsy studies show that half of all persons over the age of sixty have significant coronary artery disease, although it may not have caused symptoms or obvious problems.

♥ Heart failure is the most common cause of hospitalization for persons sixty-five and older. In particular, diastolic heart failure, which is due to a stiffening of the left ventricle—the heart's main pumping chamber—is more common in the elderly but uncommon in the young. It's important to recognize this difference because treatment for diastolic heart failure will differ markedly from therapy for other, more common causes of heart failure. Elderly women with heart failure outnumber men, perhaps because they are more likely to have high blood pressure and other problems associated with an increased risk of heart failure.

♥ About 50 percent of Americans aged sixty to sixty-nine have high blood pressure and after age seventy, 75 percent are hypertensive; these people face an increased risk of heart attacks, heart failure, and stroke. Even in younger people, systolic blood pressure (the higher of the two numbers in a blood pressure reading) is a more potent predictor of a heart attack or other cardiovascular event than is the diastolic pressure (the lower number)—but this is especially true in older people and systolic blood pressure characteristically rises in the elderly. In this regard, ongoing studies document the importance of lowering systolic blood pressure, something we once thought was unnecessary.

♥ Enlargement and/or thickening of the left ventricle, the heart's main pumping chamber, becomes increasingly common with advancing age, indicating increased risk of clinical heart failure.

♥ Age-related changes in metabolism and the arteries, a rise in blood cholesterol, an increased risk of diabetes, and increases in fibrinogen and other clotting factors can accelerate development of atherosclerosis, the buildup of fatty deposits in the arteries. In turn, atherosclerosis increases the risk of a heart attack.

♥ By age sixty-five, three in four Americans have at least one chronic disease that can complicate the treatment of coexisting heart disease. These disorders include arthritis and other orthopedic problems, diabetes, kidney and liver problems, and, especially among those over eighty, memory problems and dementia.

♥ Age-related metabolic changes, including decreased kidney and liver function, alter an older person's response to medications and increase the risk of adverse drug reactions.

DIAGNOSING HEART DISEASE IN THE ELDERLY

Diagnostic studies in the elderly are much the same as those for younger patients, although some adjustments may be necessary. For example, a frail elderly person or one with severe arthritis may be unable to undergo a treadmill exercise stress test, but can be given a drug to increase the heart rate and widen (dilate) the coronary arteries, thereby mimicking exercise and achieving the desired objective when performed in conjunction with either echocardiography or nuclear imaging. Angiography and other invasive examinations may carry a small added risk, but with proper precautions can be carried out (see Chapter 6).

LIFESTYLE AND PREVENTIVE MEASURES

Some people think that preventive measures and aggressive treatment are of little or limited value in the elderly. They couldn't be more wrong. Even the frail elderly benefit from exercise and cardiovascular fitness training, even though an appropriate regimen may differ from that prescribed for a younger person. Numerous studies show that even the very old—people over the age of eighty-five or ninety—who engage in regular exercise and moderate weight training can enjoy increased strength, mobility, balance, and enhanced well-being. The exercise program should be designed by a physician, physical therapist, or exercise physiologist and tailored to meet individual needs. Cross training can be especially beneficial in the elderly because it minimizes the risk of overuse injuries. (For more on exercise and heart disease, see Chapter 2.)

Similarly, nutrition is an often neglected factor in improving the health of the elderly. Many older people lack the resources and incentives to prepare meals that offer a variety of vegetables, fruits, whole grains, lean meats, and other dietary components recommended for good health. Instead, elderly persons—especially those who live alone and have limited incomes—subsist on foods like toast, tea, canned soups (generally high in salt, low in fiber), sweets, and convenience meals that don't require preparation or even refrigeration. Such diets exacerbate many of the problems linked to heart disease and aging, especially diabetes, obesity, high blood pressure, and constipation. Resources exist to minimize these problems, but unfortunately, the problem often does not get the attention or funding it deserves. Still, help may be forthcoming from programs like Meals on Wheels, which delivers nutritious meals to disabled or homebound persons, and senior centers and area Offices for the Aging, which provide free or low-cost meals as well as other services.

CARDIOVASCULAR MEDICATIONS

Drug therapy is a mainstay of treatment of heart disease in both the elderly and the young, but aging affects dosages, the risk of adverse reactions, and drug interactions. As people age, their ability to metabolize and use medications changes. For example, an appropriate drug and dosage of an antihypertensive medication for a young person may pose myriad problems for an older person. In addition, many older people who have multiple chronic disorders take medications to treat each, and these various drugs can interact with each other. So it is especially important to check all of a patient's medications, including over-the-counter products and alternative remedies—when prescribing any drug.

More frequent monitoring is recommended for elderly patients, especially those who are taking a number of medications. For example, a common regimen calls for a patient to take a statin drug to lower blood cholesterol, two or three different antihypertensives to control high blood pressure, an oral diabetes medication to regulate blood sugar, and perhaps a painkiller or anti-inflammatory drug for arthritis. Add to this a variety of vitamins and minerals, an over-the-counter painkiller and sleep aid, and perhaps some herbal preparations such as St. John's wort or ginkgo biloba, and you have a recipe for drug interactions. This is why it's so important for all patients, regardless of age, to inform their doctors and pharmacists of all medications and remedies—prescription, over-the-counter, and herbal. In addition, older patients should undergo more frequent blood tests to check for possible diminished liver or kidney function, which affects dosage and the type of drug prescribed.

SURGICAL INTERVENTIONS

As illustrated by the case of John, patients in their eighties and even nineties are increasingly undergoing procedures such as coronary bypass surgery, angioplasty, and valve replacement. Just a few years ago, many doctors declined to refer very old patients for heart surgery on the premise that the risks outweighed any potential benefits. This is no longer the case. In the United States, for example, one-fourth of all angioplasty procedures and coronary bypass operations are performed in patients over age seventy-five. Thanks to improved surgical techniques and a generally healthier older population, many doctors now recommend surgical treatment for even their oldest patients. In particular, aortic stenosis is very common among the very elderly. One exception to this trend involves heart transplant surgery, which generally is not done in patients over age seventy on the assumption that younger persons will benefit more from receiving one of the very few donor organs available.

ECONOMIC CONSIDERATIONS

The increased treatment options for heart patients, especially the elderly, inevitably raise the question of who will pay. There's no doubt that providing optimal care can be costly, and burgeoning health-care costs are a national concern. Medicare picks up the tab for most physician visits, diagnostic tests, hospitalizations, and surgeries for elderly patients, but it does not necessarily cover medications, which can cost several hundred dollars a month. Private insurance and the recently enacted Medicare drug coverage may help, but patients may find they still face high bills with little help in paying them. Elderly persons on fixed incomes may face difficult choices when it comes to paying for expensive medications. There are, however, avenues of help. Many drug companies offer low-cost or even free medications for needy patients. Ask your doctor or check with the pharmaceutical manufacturer. Also, many doctors and clinics give needy patients free drug samples when they are available.

Other strategies can help defray the cost of prescription drugs. Ask your doctor about generic alternatives or even older medications, which can be just as effective but less costly than newer, highly promoted drugs. Also check whether you are eligible for union or veteran's drug benefits. Some states, too, have instituted plans to purchase collectively lower-cost medications for their employees and Medicaid recipients. In addition, you might ask your doctor about pill splitting. For example, if you take thirty milligrams of an antihypertensive drug, a sixty-milligram pill may cost the same or only pennies more. The higher-dose pill can be split (some pharmacists will do this for you, or you can buy a low-cost pill-splitting device) to double the number of dosages you can get from a single prescription.

THE ISSUE OF COMPLIANCE

Obviously, any medical regimen can achieve its goals only if it is followed faithfully—something often easier said than done. Numerous studies have found that half or more of all patients on multiple drug regimens do not use their medications as directed. There are many reasons for this, but one of the most common is simply forgetting to take medications according to the prescribed schedule. This problem is especially common among older people who may be taking a number of different medications and have memory problems. Even those whose memory is intact may simply forget to take a medication or take an overdose because they can't remember whether they've taken a drug and then repeat the dosage just to be sure.

Such problems are easily remedied by putting medications in a pill counter or tracker. These devices are readily available in pharmacies (some pharmacists will even set it up for you) and are designed to avoid medication errors. One of the more popular models holds up to a month's supply, with a compartment for each day of the week. Others are designed to aid people who must take medications at different times of the day; for example, they may contain compartments for drugs taken in the morning, midday, evening, and at bedtime. Some have alarms that ring at the times when medication should be taken. Whatever type you choose, keep it in a convenient place where it can serve as a reminder to take your medication. Although pill counters are easy to use, at times it may be necessary for a family member or caregiver to set them up for an elderly person. Also, devise some sort of reminder—for example, an alarm or calendar—for liquid medication, those requiring refrigeration, or other products that can't be put in a pill counter.

SUMMING UP

The elderly make up the largest proportion of heart patients, and cardiovascular disease is the leading cause of death among Americans over age sixty-five. Even so, heart disease is not an inevitable part of aging; the human heart is designed to last a lifetime, and even the very elderly can benefit from lifestyle changes and other preventive approaches. When heart disease does develop, diagnosis and appropriate treatment can minimize its harmful effects and lead to a longer, healthier life.

11

Heart Disease in Minority Populations

The U.S. population, with its great racial, ethnic, and cultural diversity, is often likened to a human melting pot. Each year, the population balance shifts. Today, people of African, Hispanic, Asian, and Native American background comprise about 30 percent of the U.S. population; by the year 2050, this proportion is expected to grow to almost 50 percent.

Until very recently, many assumed that as minority groups became assimilated into the population at large, their health problems would mirror those of the majority. But in the area of cardiovascular disease, this has not always been the case. Some minority groups appear to be especially vulnerable to cardiovascular disease, and in general, these diseases exact a higher toll from minority groups than from the majority white population. The discrepancies are often blamed on economic factors and poor access to health care services, and these factors certainly play a significant role. But they do not fully explain why certain groups are disproportionately afflicted: instead, it appears that both genetic and cultural differences may be involved.

CARDIOVASCULAR DISEASE AMONG AFRICAN AMERICANS

Although cardiovascular disease is relatively rare in Africa itself, African Americans suffer a higher incidence of it when compared to their white counterparts. When cardiovascular disease strikes African Americans, they are less likely to survive a heart attack or stroke, and medications that work well in whites are less effective in blacks. Specific differences include:

High Blood Pressure

About 30 percent of African Americans have high blood pressure, and for those who do have it, their high blood pressure also tends to be more severe and more resistant to treatment than the same disease in whites. This difference in large part accounts for the higher death rate from heart attacks and strokes among African Americans. Some researchers have theorized that a genetic predisposition to conserve salt is a factor. The typical African American diet is high in salt and low in potassium and calcium (minerals that may help control blood pressure). Further confirming the theory is the fact that salt restriction and treatment with diuretics, which remove excess salt and fluid from the body, are very effective in lowering blood pressure in this group, more so than in whites.

Coronary Artery Disease

African Americans have the world's highest death rate from heart attacks and other manifestations of coronary artery disease. The African American survival rate from heart attacks is much lower than that of whites and Asian Americans. The reasons for this difference are complex, but undoubtedly involve disparities in health care, economic factors, social and psychological issues, and perhaps genetics.

Stroke

The number of strokes and the stroke death rate among African Americans are also much higher than those of other population groups, presumably due to their increased incidence of high blood pressure. Stroke also occurs at an earlier age among African Americans than among whites, and a stroke is four times more likely to cause death in a black patient than in a white patient. The toll is highest in the so-called stroke belt of the southeastern United States, where high blood pressure and obesity are also the most prevalent.

Obesity

African Americans have a much higher incidence of obesity, defined as a body mass index (BMI) of thirty or higher, than other population groups. Obesity is especially prevalent among African American women, who weigh an average of seventeen pounds more than their white counterparts. Throughout the South, where hypertension and stroke are especially common among minority groups, more than 70 percent of African American women are obese. Obesity itself increases the risk of a heart attack; it also contributes to high blood cholesterol, diabetes, and metabolic syndrome (insulin resistance combined with high blood pressure, obesity, and high blood lipids).

Diabetes

More than 18 percent of African Americans suffer from diabetes (compared to 11 percent of white Americans). Diabetes is a major—and growing—risk factor for heart attacks, strokes, and kidney failure among all Americans. But African Americans, as well as Hispanics, are afflicted more often and more severely than whites. The differences are attributed to diet, sedentary lifestyle, and perhaps a genetic predisposition. In addition, diabetes often goes undiagnosed and untreated in minority populations until it is at an advanced stage and has caused permanent damage to vital organs.

Left Ventricular Thickening and Heart Failure

African Americans lead other population groups in heart failure. The increased incidence of an enlarged and thickened (hypertrophic) left ventricle, the heart's main pumping chamber, begins at an early age in this group. The causes are not fully understood, but the predominance of hypertension among African Americans is a major contributing factor. Over time, the enlarged, thickened heart muscle weakens and is unable to pump enough blood to meet the body's needs—a characteristic of heart failure.

CARDIOVASCULAR DISEASE AMONG HISPANIC AMERICANS

Patterns of cardiovascular disease among Hispanics vary according to country of origin, and are somewhat puzzling. For example, Hispanic Americans tend to have a lower incidence of high blood pressure when compared to white Americans and other population groups. But they still have a higher-than-average death rate from cardiovascular disease and stroke. Among specific differences are the following:

High Blood Pressure

About 14 percent of Hispanic Americans have high blood pressure—a percentage much lower than that of African Americans and non-Hispanic whites. Within the Hispanic community, Puerto Ricans have the highest incidence of hypertension, followed by Cubans and Mexican Americans. When hypertension develops, it tends to be more resistant to treatment than hypertension in other population groups.

Coronary Artery Disease

Although the incidence of coronary artery disease among Hispanics has increased in recent decades, it is still less than that of other population groups.

Obesity

Hispanics have a high incidence of overweight and obesity, with a mean BMI of twenty-eight (anything over twenty-five or twenty-six is classified as overweight), which is only slightly lower than that of African Americans.

Diabetes

Hispanics lead other minority groups in the incidence of diabetes, although the death rate from this disease is somewhat higher among African Americans. More than 20 percent of Hispanic Americans over the age of forty have diabetes, and of these, 70 percent also have high blood pressure—a lower percentage than that of African Americans, but still high enough to greatly increase the risk of heart attacks and stroke, as well as kidney failure and other serious complications of the disease.

Metabolic Syndrome

Although Hispanics have a very high incidence of insulin resistance and diabetes, they are somewhat less likely than African Americans to develop the high blood pressure component of metabolic syndrome.

CARDIOVASCULAR DISEASE AMONG NATIVE AMERICANS

There's no doubt that the health of Native Americans has suffered greatly as they have tried to adapt to modern life in the United States. Even those who are not beset by poverty, alcohol and drug abuse, and social isolation tend to fare poorly. This is especially true in the area of diabetes and some forms of cardiovascular disease. Diabetes—once rare among Native Americans—is now endemic among the Navaho and some other Native Americans of the West. It is thought that a genetic predisposition plays a role, exacerbated by obesity attributed to a high-fat diet and sedentary lifestyle. Coronary artery disease and high blood pressure are also increasingly common among Native Americans, resulting in an increased incidence of heart attacks and strokes.

CARDIOVASCULAR DISEASE AMONG PEOPLE OF SOUTH ASIAN ORIGIN

As the number of Americans with origins in India, Pakistan, and other countries of the Indian subcontinent grows, we are becoming increasingly aware of their cardiovascular problems. Chief among these is a type of rapidly advancing coronary artery disease that is resistant to conventional treatments and somewhat different from that seen in white Americans. Anatomically, the disease tends to be very diffuse and involve the entire length of the coronary arteries. It also tends to run in families, especially those with insulin resistance. Weight does not appear to be as important a determining factor in this population group; even those who are of normal weight are often afflicted. Ongoing studies are seeking reasons for these differences.

IMPLICATIONS FOR TREATMENT

Clearly ethnicity, race, and cultural background all play important roles in the development and treatment of cardiovascular disease. We are learning, for example, that African Americans are likely to benefit more from some types of antihypertensive drugs, such as diuretics and calcium channel blockers, than from beta blockers, ACE inhibitors, and ARBs. We also know that heart failure tends to be more common, and exhibit different symptoms, in African Americans than other population groups, and may require more aggressive and different therapy involving vasodilator medications and nitrates.

Ethnicity and cultural differences, as well as a language barrier, may also pose special challenges for tackling obesity, tobacco use, and a lack of physical activity. For patients struggling to communicate or feeling resistant to changes that don't seem to fit their native culture, intensive counseling and peer group support are often critical to the success of a long-term treatment program. Given today's economic constraints, some health-care providers question the need for and viability of such efforts. But funds used for this kind of early support and education are very well spent. It is much more expensive to treat advanced heart disease or care for patients who have suffered a stroke, amputation, kidney failure, or other ravages of an undiagnosed or undertreated cardiac disorder.

SUMMING UP

Even after becoming assimilated into the general population, many minority groups harbor risk factors that make them more vulnerable to certain forms of cardiovascular disease. These group-specific risk factors must be considered in any evaluation and treatment. Some populations may also be hampered by social and economic factors, including reduced access to preventive health care. Addressing these issues early and well is not just an ethical imperative; in those cases where a minority patient is unable to find adequate care without assistance, education and other supports help to avoid higher costs for all down the road.

CHAPTER

12

Young Athletes and Heart Disease

A
thletes of all ages occupy a unique place in our culture. They are thought
of as the very paragons of health. Collegiate and professional athletes are
idolized by society both on and off the playing field or court. Indeed, it
is hard for us to understand the existence of heart disease and sudden cardiac
death in such individuals. Yet every year we hear about sudden cardiac death in
young or relatively young athletes. How could an all-American basketball player
suddenly drop dead on the court? These events often make nationwide headlines
and raise concern about the safety of organized sports programs.

The problem is hardly new. One of history's most celebrated cases occurred
more than 2,500 years ago when Pheidippides, the Athenian long-distance runner,
dropped dead after running more than twenty-six miles from the battlefield at
Marathon to Athens to announce victory of the Greeks. When compared to
other forms of cardiovascular mortality, however, the numbers of such incidents
in the United States today are very small—about three hundred deaths a year
among athletes, representing only a tiny fraction of the 10 to 15 million Americans of all ages who participate in organized sports. A survey in Minnesota placed
the risk for high school athletes in organized sports at one in 200,000, and the
American Heart Association says this ratio can be extrapolated to the nation as
a whole. Older athletes (such as middle-aged marathoners) have a somewhat
higher risk; but in this group the underlying cause is often previously undetected
coronary artery disease. Consequently, while we need to be aware of exercise-

related deaths in young, physically fit, and apparently healthy athletes, it is truly an unusual occurrence.

CAUSES OF CARDIAC DEATH IN YOUNG ATHLETES

Undetected preexisting heart disease causes most of the exercise-related sudden deaths in young athletes. Other noncardiac causes include asthma, heatstroke, and drug abuse, which are not discussed here. In most instances, the cardiac cause goes undetected during life, although in retrospect the majority of individuals—some studies put the figure at 80 percent—have experienced some warning symptoms. The most common cardiac abnormalities leading to sudden death include:

Hypertrophic Cardiomyopathy

An inherited condition, hypertrophic cardiomyopathy (HCM) is characterized by an overgrowth of heart muscle cells leading to thickening of the heart chambers' walls. HCM is also associated with abnormal cardiac arrhythmias, and it is the leading cause of sudden cardiac deaths in young athletes in the United States.

Coronary Artery Anomalies

Congenital abnormalities of the coronary artery are generally considered the second leading cause of sudden death. In one of the most common anomalies, one of the coronary arteries arises from the wrong side of the aorta. For example, the left coronary artery may arise from the right side of the aorta, close to the origin of the right coronary artery. The path taken by this abnormal artery places extra physical stress on the heart, which can result in a serious, even life-threatening problem under certain circumstances.

Chest Trauma

Unlike other causes of sudden cardiac death, chest trauma (commotio cordis), which most commonly happens to children and adolescents, does not involve any structural heart disease. Instead, it results from a blunt, nonpenetrating blow to the chest that produces a fatal cardiac arrhythmia (ventricular fibrillation) even though it does not cause structural damage to the heart itself. Typically, the trauma producing the fatal arrhythmia is not unusual for the specific sport. The most common examples include blows to the chest from a baseball or hockey puck, collisions between athletes, or a direct hit to the chest during participation in a martial arts sport such as karate.

Myocarditis

Myocarditis, which involves inflammation of the heart muscle, is often caused by a viral infection. As a result of the infection and inflammation, the heart becomes enlarged and often functions poorly; myocarditis may also disturb the heart's rhythm. An athlete who is unaware of the problem can suffer serious consequences, including sudden death, during intense exercise and competition.

Arrhythmias Caused by Right Ventricular Cardiomyopathy

A condition that involves enlargement of the right ventricle, arrhythmias caused by right ventricular cardiomyopathy are uncommon in the United States, but have been cited as the most common cause of death among athletes in northern Italy. The reason for this geographic discrepancy is unknown. Death is caused by cardiac rhythm disturbances originating in the right ventricle, which also may not function normally.

Ruptured Aortic Aneurysm from Marfan Syndrome

Marfan syndrome is a genetic disease affecting the body's connective tissue. It is characterized by a specific physical appearance that includes increased height, abnormally long bones, and excessive joint flexibility. (Some observers speculate that Abraham Lincoln had Marfan syndrome, but this is based more on his appearance than any medical data.) People with Marfan syndrome may have vision problems as well as blood vessel abnormalities that may result in an aneurysm (outward bulging) of the aorta—the body's largest artery that arises from the heart and carries blood into the body's circulation. Sudden death occurs in athletes when a large aortic aneurysm ruptures.

Electrocardiographic Conditions Associated with Sudden Death

There are two electrocardiographic conditions associated with sudden death, Brugada syndrome and Long QT syndrome, that are diagnosed only by specific abnormalities detected by an electrocardiogram (ECG). Both conditions are inherited and, consequently, a family history of either justifies testing to detect them in a young athlete. Both conditions can result in sudden cardiac death due to a fatal ventricular arrhythmia.

Other Conditions

A number of other rare conditions can result in sudden cardiac death in athletes. These include a narrowing or stiffening of the aortic valve (aortic stenosis), undiagnosed premature coronary artery disease, and unspecific cardiomyopathy (an enlargement and weakening of the heart chambers, or ventricles).

VARIABLES TO BE CONSIDERED

In the United States, football and basketball are the most common sports associated with sudden cardiac death. Not surprisingly, because of cultural preferences in Europe, soccer is the most common sport linked to the sudden death of participants. Gender may play a role. Although sudden death occasionally occurs in women—the case of Flo Hyman, the Olympic volleyball star, comes to mind—male athletes who die suddenly outnumber females nine to one. Race may also be a factor. For example, most of the athletes who die of hypertrophic cardiomyopathy are African American, even though this condition is diagnosed more often in Caucasians. The reason for this discrepancy is unknown.

APPROACHES TO SCREENING YOUNG ATHLETES

Screening for previously unrecognized cardiovascular disorders in athletes before they participate in their sport—whether through physically examining the athlete or through taking a history of any such disorders in family members—can alert a doctor to a potentially fatal condition. But there are no uniform national guidelines for screening young athletes, and standards vary greatly from state to state. In addition, universal screening is not practical: it would involve examining 10 million to 15 million young people, most of whom will be found to be basically healthy and free of heart disease.

Most high school and college athletes in the United States, then, generally are required only to have a health-care professional take a medical history and perform a basic physical examination. Under current guidelines, the medical history should include questions of any family members who suffered premature sudden cardiac death or unexplained death, as well as determining whether close relatives have developed premature heart disease (for example, a heart attack or diagnosis of serious coronary artery diseases before the age of fifty). The athlete also should be questioned specifically about a personal history of heart murmurs, high blood pressure, excessive fatigue, fainting or near fainting, shortness of breath, or chest discomfort.

The physical examination should focus on detecting any heart murmurs, altered pulses in the lower extremities, high blood pressure, or the physical appearance that may point to Marfan syndrome. Any abnormal findings should lead to further examinations, including, where appropriate, an electrocardiogram, echocardiogram, Holter monitor, tilt-table testing, or magnetic resonance imaging (MRI). These tests, described more fully in Chapter 6, are designed to identify any significant heart conditions that could result in sudden cardiac death during athletic participation and other activities.

RECOMMENDATIONS FOR YOUNG ATHLETES

Over the last five years, a number of school districts have mandated that automated external defibrillators (AEDs) be made available in gyms and at sporting events. While AEDs may be useful in saving an athlete who suffers a cardiac arrest, they are not sufficient protection against sudden cardiac events in athletes with known cardiac disease. Thus, when an abnormality is identified we must ask, Would this risk be reduced if the athlete stopped training or competing?

These and other questions were addressed at the Thirty-sixth Bethesda Conference on Eligibility Recommendations for Competitive Athletes with Cardiovascular Abnormalities. The detailed report that came out of the 2004 conference defines our current state of knowledge regarding the relative risk of a variety of conditions. In particular, athletes with the following disorders should not participate in competitive organized sports:

- ♥ Hypertrophic cardiomyopathy (even if under treatment)
- ♥ Coronary artery anomalies
- ♥ Myocarditis (a reevaluation six months after the end of the infection can determine whether there's been sufficient recovery to allow a return to sports)
- ♥ Marfan syndrome
- ♥ Inherited cardiac rhythm disorders such as Long QT syndrome and Brugada syndrome

OTHER VARIABLES TO CONSIDER

A number of other forms of heart disease can occur in young athletes, including congenital defects, valvular defects, and miscellaneous cardiovascular abnormalities, must be evaluated individually. As a general rule, athletes with mild forms of these conditions often can participate in some organized sports, whereas those with more advanced forms of disease should not. Decisions concerning participation, however, should be made together with a qualified health-care professional.

Treatment of diagnosed cardiovascular disorders also plays a role in determining an appropriate activity for a young athlete. For example, a number of cardiovascular conditions that afflict young adults may be treated with beta blocking medications, which may cause fatigue and hinder athletic performance.

Obviously, all sports cannot be lumped together when considering the appropriateness of participation. For example, bowling makes fewer physical demands than does martial arts, long-distance running, or basketball. Consequently, relatively relaxed sports may well be appropriate for certain individuals with known cardiac conditions. For example, a person with Marfan syndrome may be able to engage in bowling or golf, whereas basketball and other endurance sports are off-limits. Before selecting a sports activity, you must discuss the options in detail with a cardiologist with expertise in this area.

"ATHLETE'S HEART"

Consistent training in endurance sports, such as running, or isometric activities, such as weight lifting, can produce changes in the heart's structure. These changes, often referred to as the "athlete's heart," are not associated with increased risk. Athletic training can produce a modest increase in heart wall thickness—a condition called benign ventricular hypertrophy—as well as an increase in heart size or volume. Isometric activities are associated mostly with increased ventricular wall thickness and less of an increase in the size of the ventricles. In contrast, endurance sport training is associated more with an increase in heart size and less with an effect on wall thickness. In athletes there may also be changes in the resting electrocardiogram that are consistent with athlete's heart and do not necessarily indicate an underlying serious heart condition.

SUMMING UP

Although relatively rare, undetected cardiovascular disease can cause sudden cardiac death in young athletes. A careful physical examination and medical history can help identify athletes who are at risk and who may benefit from more detailed evaluation and testing. Recognizing the presence of such a cardiac condition should lead to further recommendations concerning the suitability of participation in competitive sports and the type of sport most appropriate for the young person. It is important to recognize, too, that well-trained athletes often will experience changes in their heart structure that can be detected on an electrocardiogram; these do not indicate an underlying serious heart condition.

13

Adults with Congenital Heart Disease

Congenital heart disease is an abnormality of the heart's structure or function that is present at birth. The malformations, which develop in the fetus, are often detected before or at birth, or shortly thereafter—occasionally, they show up much later in adult life. Congenital heart defects are relatively rare, occurring in only about one of every hundred live births, and just 15 percent of these result in serious or complex heart disease. Moreover, the tremendous improvements in medical and surgical techniques over the past thirty years now enable many patients with even complex congenital heart disease to survive into adult life. Consequently, for the first time the number of adults with congenital heart disease now equals that of children with these disorders. While the true incidence of congenital cardiovascular malformations is somewhat difficult to determine, in 2000 there were about 485,000 adults with moderately to very complex congenital heart disease and an additional 300,000 individuals with simpler forms of the condition.

As more children born with these heart defects survive into adulthood, treating the condition becomes an increasingly important medical issue. The myriad issues facing these patients were highlighted at the Thirty-second Bethesda Conference, "Care of the Adult with Congenital Heart Disease," held in October 2000. The report of that conference, published in April 2001 (see Further Reading and Resources), stressed the complexity and technical difficulties posed in treating these patients. This chapter focuses on some of the more general issues outlined in the report.

A BROAD PICTURE OF CONGENITAL HEART DISEASE

All parts of the heart can be affected by congenital cardiac malformations, which can occur alone or in combination with other abnormalities. For example, each of the four heart valves may be malformed, resulting in either narrowing and stiffening (valvular stenosis) or widening (dilation), and in turn causing a back-flow of blood (regurgitation). Narrowing or stiffening of the pulmonic or aortic valves can also exist at levels above and below the valves, conditions referred to as supravalvular and subvalvular stenosis, respectively.

Some congenital defects cause abnormal openings in the wall (septum) between the heart's lower chambers (the left and right ventricles), resulting in a ventricular septal defect. When the abnormal openings occur between the upper chambers (the left and right atria), the condition is called an atrial septal defect. Other conditions may result in high blood pressure in the lungs (pulmonary hypertension).

In some of the more severe types of congenital heart disease, the patient's skin may have a bluish cast (cyanosis) because of inadequate oxygen in the circulating blood. Another complex form of congenital disease involves an abnormal rotation of the heart and blood vessels in which the major arteries are attached to the wrong ventricles. Each of these and other abnormalities presents varying challenges that must be addressed and treated according to individual needs.

SEVERITY OF CONGENITAL HEART DISEASE

Patients with congenital heart disease are grouped into three categories, depending on the complexity and severity of the condition; these are listed in Box 19. (We have not attempted to define the conditions here; instead, the list is intended to make you aware of where specific diseases fit in the overall spectrum of severity.) Proper classification becomes very important in selecting the type and location of medical care. For example, if you have "simple" congenital heart disease, you generally can be managed by a cardiologist in your community. If the disease is of "moderate severity" or "great complexity," however, you will likely require treatment in a regional referral center that offers multidisciplinary teams of caregivers (see Box 20).

Box 19

CLASSES OF CONGENITAL HEART DISEASES

Simple Congenital Heart Disease

Native Disease (Conditions That Have Not Been Treated Surgically)

- Isolated congenital aortic valve disease
- Isolated congenital mitral valve disease
- Isolated patent foramen ovale or small atrial septal defect
- Isolated small ventricular septal defect
- Mild pulmonic stenosis

Repaired Conditions (Conditions That Have Been Treated Surgically)

- Repaired ductus arteriosus
- Repaired atrial septal defect without residual problems
- Repaired ventricular septal defect without residual problems

Congenital Heart Disease of Moderate Severity

- Aorta–left ventricular fistula
- Anomalous pulmonary venous drainage
- Atrioventricular septal defects
- Coarctation of the aorta
- Ebstein anomaly
- Subvalvular pulmonic stenosis
- Complex atrial septal defect (ostium primum)
- Patent ductus arteriosus
- Pulmonary valve regurgitation (moderate to severe)
- Pulmonary valve stenosis (moderate to severe)
- Sinus of Valsalva fistula/aneurysm
- Sinus venosus atrial septal defect
- Subvalvular or supravalvular aortic stenosis

(*continued*)

(Box 19 *continued*)

- Tetralogy of Fallot
- Ventricular septal defect with associated conditions

Congenital Heart Disease of Great Complexity

- Conduits, valved or nonvalved (resulting from surgical treatment)
- Cyanotic congenital heart disease of all forms
- Double outlet ventricle
- Eisenmenger syndrome
- Fontan procedure (surgical treatment)
- Mitral atresia
- Single ventricle
- Pulmonary atresia
- Pulmonary vascular obstructive disease
- Transposition of the great arteries
- Tricuspid atresia
- Truncus arteriosus

Modified from Thirty-second Bethesda Conference, "Care of the Adult with Congenital Heart Disease," *Journal of the American College of Cardiology* 37 (2001): 1161.

Some forms of congenital heart disease can be cured surgically; in other circumstances, however, surgery may be performed only to relieve symptoms, or to correct some of the problems without actually producing a cure. Box 19 distinguishes between conditions in which there has been surgical repair (repaired) and those that have not been treated surgically (native).

SIMILARITIES TO OTHER FORMS OF HEART DISEASE

Patients with congenital heart disease often experience many of the same problems faced by patients with other forms of heart disease (see Chapter 7). One of these is heart failure, in which the heart cannot pump enough blood to meet the body's needs. The problem can involve either or both of the ventricles; there may also be a marked thickening (hypertrophy) of either of these pumping chambers.

Congenital heart disease can also result in abnormal electrical pathways in the heart, resulting in disturbances in the heart's normal rhythm. Specific types of congenital heart disease have a propensity for specific types of rhythm disturbance. The more common examples include supraventricular arrhythmias, which arise in the heart chambers above the ventricle, or ventricular arrhythmias, which arise in the ventricles themselves.

In the condition known as pulmonary hypertension, the blood pressure in the lungs' pulmonary arteries is too high. Although patients with other forms of severe heart disease often may develop pulmonary hypertension, the condition involves a different mechanism in patients with congenital heart disease. Specifically, in congenital heart disease the pulmonary hypertension develops in response to increased blood flow through the lungs. Successful treatment relates to the severity and duration of the high blood pressure in the pulmonary arteries.

UNIQUE MEDICAL ISSUES

While adults with congenital heart defects face many of the same problems as patients whose disorders developed later in life, there are several aspects of treatment that are unique to congenital disease. Most congenital abnormalities are discovered early in life, for example, so patients need to be aware that when they approach age eighteen, they should switch doctors—from a pediatric cardiologist to one who treats adults. Your pediatric cardiologist may be able to refer you to such a doctor; in many instances, these specialists collaborate with the referring pediatrician, at least during the transitional phase.

In addition, as mentioned earlier, patients with some types of congenital heart disease may have a bluish tinge to their skin, or cyanosis, indicating inadequate oxygen levels in the blood. This condition can cause an increase in red blood cells, resulting in abnormally thick blood. Sometimes this problem is treated with periodic removal of blood (phlebotomy). Patients with cyanosis may also develop gout and arthritic joints, which require separate treatment.

Surgery unrelated to the heart may be more complicated and dangerous for patients with moderate to severe congenital heart disease. Before undergoing elective surgery, consult a surgical team with expertise in dealing with patients with congenital heart disease. And in emergency situations requiring surgery, make sure the physicians are aware of the heart problem so they can take the necessary precautions.

Pregnancy poses a unique and increased risk to women with certain types of congenital heart disease. While many women with relatively minor or treatable congenital defects can safely have babies, those with more complex disease should avoid pregnancy. Discuss potential problems and options with your doctor before attempting conception. If it is clear that pregnancy poses undue risk to the woman and/or her fetus, reliable contraception is essential. In the event that a woman with congenital heart disease does conceive, she should seek an obstetrician who specializes in high-risk pregnancies. If this applies to you, your cardiologist can help you find such a doctor or medical team experienced in treating pregnant women with your particular condition.

Because some congenital heart disorders are hereditary, it's wise to seek genetic counseling to learn the risks of passing the condition to any offspring. Many congenital defects can be detected early in pregnancy using sonography or more invasive studies, such as a biopsy of fetal tissue or amniocentesis, the removal of some cells shed by the fetus into the amniotic fluid as a way of screening for certain genetic abnormalities.

Perhaps not surprisingly, patients with long-standing congenital heart disease may have psychosocial problems involving such issues as emotional health, family dynamics, financial issues, and insurance. Don't hesitate to ask your health care team about services that may assist you and your family.

TREATMENT OPTIONS

The 2000 Bethesda conference on adults with congenital heart disease stressed that patients with simple congenital heart disease can be treated by local cardiologists. Such individuals manifest few clinical problems and generally have excellent long-term outlook. Individuals with congenital heart disease of moderate or great severity or complexity, however, are likely best served by regional referral centers specifically designed to treat adults with congenital heart disease. (See Box 19 for general information on your condition's level of severity.) Such regional referral centers are developing throughout the United States and in Canada and Europe. Staffed generally by physicians who are both adult and pediatric cardiologists with expertise in specific congenital heart disorders, the centers typically have teams of physicians who also have expertise in the treatment of related problems such as cardiac arrhythmias, and are skilled in the use of cutting-edge technologies like echocardiography, magnetic resonance imaging, and other imaging techniques to diagnose complex malformations. Such centers also have physicians skilled in many other specialties, such as anesthesiology, obstetrics and gynecology, kidney disease, hematology, psychiatry and psychology, and other disciplines relevant to patients with congenital heart disease. In addi-

---

Box 20

CENTERS SPECIALIZING IN THE CARE OF ADULT PATIENTS WITH
CONGENITAL HEART DISEASE

The following list, while not complete, represents a broad geographic distribution of large centers. Your doctor can direct you to other specialists or centers.

- Boston Adult Congenital Heart (BACH) Service, Boston
- Cleveland Clinic, Cleveland, Ohio
- Children's Hospital of Philadelphia (CHOP), Philadelphia
- Columbia-Presbyterian Medical Center, New York City
- Emory University Medical Center, Atlanta
- Mayo Clinic, Rochester, Minnesota
- Northwestern University Medical Center, Evanston, Illinois
- Ohio State University Medical Center, Columbus, Ohio
- Stanford University Medical Center, Palo Alto, California
- Texas Children's Hospital, Houston
- Toronto General Hospital, Toronto, Ontario
- University of California Los Angeles (UCLA) Medical Center, Los Angeles
- University of Michigan Medical Center, Ann Arbor
- Washington University, Barnes Medical Center, St. Louis, Missouri
- Yale New Haven Medical Center, New Haven, Connecticut

---

tion, there are full-time social workers and support staff available to assist with a wide range of issues. (See Box 20 for a listing of some centers.)

SUMMING UP

Treatment of congenital heart disease in adults is an evolving field, although over the past thirty years great strides have been made in managing and curing these disorders. Consequently, children born with congenital heart disorders are now surviving into adulthood, leading to a new discipline in adult cardiology. Depending on the complexity of the condition, many patients can be treated locally. Others may benefit from seeking the expertise at large regional centers. Regardless of where treatment is given, recent advances in other areas of cardiovascular disease have greatly improved the outlook for adults with congenital heart disorders.

14

Practical Advice for Travelers

Within reason, heart patients can engage in most day-to-day activities, including work, recreational pursuits, and travel. But travel may require certain precautions, especially when it includes air travel or visiting very high altitudes. Although the occurrence of heart attacks and other significant cardiac events during air travel is relatively low, they account for as much as 10 to 20 percent of all medical incidents on airplanes. Consequently, both the airlines and the Federal Aviation Administration (FAA) have taken steps to minimize the cardiovascular risk of air travel. There are also a number of precautions that individuals can take.

AIR TRAVEL

Generally speaking, most heart patients can safely travel by air, but there are exceptions. You should not fly if:

- ♥ You have suffered a heart attack within the past two weeks.
- ♥ You have unstable angina—chest pains that occur during rest or under other unpredictable circumstances.
- ♥ You have undergone angioplasty or coronary stent placement within the previous two weeks.
- ♥ You have had coronary artery bypass surgery within the previous three weeks.

💜 You have poorly controlled heart failure.

💜 You suffer from serious heart rhythm disorders, specifically uncontrolled ventricular or supraventricular arrhythmias.

Oxygen Needs

Anyone who has ever taken a commercial airline flight has undoubtedly watched an attendant demonstrate the use of an oxygen mask in case of an emergency, yet these devices are very rarely needed. Airline cabins are pressurized to provide a comfortable environment for normal breathing. They are not pressurized to sea level, however, which results in a modest but real decrease in the oxygen content of passengers' blood. For most people, this is not a problem; exceptions may include passengers with heart or lung disorders. In addition, air travel, particularly after the September 11 terrorist attacks, may provoke anxiety. The combination of reduced oxygen, along with increased stress, can pose special dangers to persons with coronary artery disease, resulting in chest pain or even a heart attack. Most planes carry portable supplemental oxygen; don't hesitate to request it if you have any difficulty breathing, experience chest pains, or feel any other heart-related symptoms.

If you need supplemental oxygen at sea level, you will also require it during your flight. Alert the airline to your needs well in advance of your trip and have a letter of medical clearance from your physician.

Emergency Equipment

Since 2004, the FAA has required airlines to carry at least one automatic external defibrillator (AED) on most commercial passenger planes, specifically those capable of carrying more than 7,500 pounds and that have at least one flight attendant on board. These portable defibrillators are easy to use, and all crew members are now trained to respond to cardiac-arrest emergencies. Most airports also have defibrillators in waiting rooms and other public spaces. Although these devices are not needed very often, they already have saved the lives of a number of passengers who suffered a cardiac arrest while on the plane or in an airport.

Reducing Your Risk of Blood Clots

Air travelers have an increased risk of deep venous thrombosis, the formation of blood clots in the veins of the inner legs. These can become deadly if a portion of the clot (an embolus) travels through the veins to the heart, lungs, or brain. Factors contributing to deep venous thrombosis include a pooling of blood in the legs (venous stasis) from sitting still for long periods, fluid retention, dehydration, and possibly the lowered level of blood oxygen. Although even healthy young people can develop deep venous thrombosis, the risk is especially high for heart patients and the elderly. All air travelers, regardless of age or level of risk, should move around frequently while in the air, avoid excess alcohol, and drink substantial amounts of water, juice, or other nonalcoholic beverages. To minimize the possibility of developing blood clots, follow these precautions according to your level of risk, described briefly below.* If you are unsure of your risk level, or need further information, consult your doctor.

Low Risk

Low-risk air travel is less than eight hours for a person without risk factors. To minimize risk, get up and move about every hour or so, drink plenty of water, and consider wearing below-the-knee support (compression) stockings.

Moderate Risk

You are considered to be at moderate risk when your flight is longer than eight hours and you are either older than fifty or are of any age and have large varicose veins, congestive heart failure, or decreased heart function, or are taking hormone replacement therapy. If you fall into any of these groups, minimize your risk by wearing below-the-knee compression stockings, flexing your leg muscles and walking about frequently, drinking plenty of water, and if possible, sitting in an aisle seat that allows you to stretch your legs and get up often. Some doctors also recommend aspirin therapy for moderate-risk travelers (if they are not already taking aspirin), although there are no firm data that this helps.

High Risk

High-risk air travel is defined as a flight longer than eight hours undertaken by someone who has a history of venous thromboembolism, congestive heart fail-

*Modified from S. E. Possick and M. Barry, "Evaluations and Management of the Cardiovascular Patient Embarking on Air Travel," *Annals of Internal Medicine* 141 (2004): 148–154.

ure, or decreased heart function, or has had a recent major operation such as hip or knee surgery. If any of these risk factors apply to you, minimize your risk by wearing full-length compression stockings, requesting an aisle seat, getting up and walking about frequently, and, when seated, stretching and flexing your legs at least every thirty to sixty minutes and drinking plenty of water. A preflight injection of heparin, a blood-thinning medication that helps prevent blood clots, may also be advisable.

Precautions for Persons with Pacemakers or Implanted Defibrillators (ICDs)

Air travel does not interfere with implanted pacemakers or ICDs, but these devices may set off security metal detectors. (The same is true of artificial knee joints and other implanted metal prostheses, but not of coronary stents.) If you have any of these devices, you should carry a card identifying the type of device implanted.

Although there are no reports that this has ever happened, theoretically being screened with a handheld metal detector or wand could interfere with an ICD and result in an inadvertent shock. Consequently, patients with ICDs should request a hand search if possible. If a metal-detecting wand is used, the examiner should be cautioned not to hold the magnet over the device for more than a few seconds. If it must be passed over the device more than once, at least thirty seconds should elapse between each pass.

MEDICATIONS AND MEDICAL RECORDS

When traveling, always take an ample supply of all medications in your carry-on baggage; do not pack it in your checked luggage, which may be lost or delayed. Any injectables such as insulin syringes should be clearly labeled with a professional label. All travelers should also carry an updated medication list.

Heart patients should also carry a baseline electrocardiogram, particularly if it is abnormal. If you suffer from episodes of chest pains (angina), be sure to carry a supply of nitroglycerine with you at all times. If you have an implanted device such as a pacemaker or ICD, you should carry a card with the manufacturer and device type as well as your local physician contact information.

If you are going abroad or planning an extended stay away from home, it's a good idea to have your doctor write extra prescriptions for you that can be filled at local pharmacies. Many drugs that require a prescription in the United States are available without one abroad, but don't count on this. Also, some foreign pharmacies require prescriptions from a local physician. Before you leave home, it's a good idea to have the name of a local doctor whom you can contact in case of an emergency. Your doctor or travel agent may be able to help you with this; hotels and consulates also can usually provide lists of local physicians, including those who speak your language. All developed countries have emergency medical services comparable to those in the United States, but find out before you leave what number you should call to access them, because this varies from one country to another.

TRAVEL TO HIGH ALTITUDES

Mountain climbers and skiers are well aware of the possible adverse effects of traveling to and exercising in high altitudes, typically defined as more than five thousand to eleven thousand feet above sea level. Most people can tolerate an altitude of five thousand feet (Denver, for example) without problems, but even healthy persons may run into trouble when they travel to Denver and then immediately head for high-mountain sightseeing, skiing, or climbing. If you have a heart problem, take special precautions. When you are at five thousand feet or higher, limit your exercise and give yourself ample time to adjust to the higher locale. Even healthy persons may start experiencing problems of altitude sickness when they go above eight thousand feet, and in these days of rapid air travel, many tourists are unaware of the potential hazards of breathing the air at high altitudes, which contains less oxygen than air at altitudes closer to sea level.

Heart patients and persons who suffer from diabetes, anemia, and kidney disease are especially vulnerable. When planning a trip to a high altitude—for example, Mexico City, Nepal, the Alps, or other high mountain ranges—check with your doctor about both the advisability of such travel and any precautions you should take.

Symptoms of Altitude Sickness

Almost everyone traveling to a high altitude will notice physical changes, including shortness of breath upon exertion, increased urination, more rapid breathing (hyperventilation), and an altered breathing pattern at night. These are usually transient and disappear as the body adjusts to the higher altitude. In contrast, symptoms associated with altitude or mountain sickness may worsen and should never be ignored. In general, altitude sickness is divided into three types:

1. Acute mountain sickness (AMS). Common symptoms include general malaise, similar to a hangover, as well as headache, fatigue, loss of appetite, and nausea. Many people also experience shortness of breath, dizziness, and disturbed sleep.

2. High-altitude pulmonary edema (HAPE), or water in the lungs. This is a more serious form of altitude sickness, requiring prompt treatment. Symptoms include increasing shortness of breath, even at rest; rattling or gurgling in the chest and a feeling of tightness or chest congestion; severe cough, which may be dry or produce sputum; extreme fatigue; a fast heartbeat, for example, a pulse of more than 110 beats a minute; and a bluish tinge of the face, lips, or nail beds.

3. High-altitude cerebral edema (HACE), or water in the brain. This is the most severe form of altitude sickness and, if untreated, can lead to death. Symptoms include a very severe headache, vomiting, an unsteady gait, mental confusion or altered mental state, and irritability. The onset of any of these symptoms mandates immediate evacuation to a lower altitude and intensive treatment to relieve the brain swelling.

Preventive Measures

If you have any medical problem that may make you more vulnerable to altitude sickness, consult your doctor about possible preventive medications, such as acetazolamide (Diamox). For most people, however, common sense and simple preventive measures will suffice:

- Give yourself time to adjust to the higher altitude. Don't start exercising immediately; instead, give yourself a day or two to adjust.
- Avoid alcoholic beverages, nicotine, tranquilizers, sleeping pills, and other drugs that depress the central nervous system.
- Drink plenty of fluids (experts recommend at least three to four quarts a day) to replace fluids lost through increased urination. Dehydration is a key component of altitude sickness.
- Eat a high-carbohydrate diet (70 percent or more of calories).
- Do not attempt to exercise alone, and make sure that everyone in the group is familiar with the warning signs and symptoms of altitude sickness. At very high altitudes, make sure that emergency medical supplies are available, such as oxygen and appropriate medications.

♥ If symptoms worsen, stop exercising. If you are skiing or climbing, descend immediately. If this is impossible, seek emergency treatment and as soon as possible, get to a lower altitude.

Studies conducted during the last decade indicate that ginkgo biloba, a popular herbal remedy, may help prevent altitude sickness. In one study involving forty volunteers who lived at a moderate altitude (less than five thousand feet), participants were divided into two groups. One received a placebo and the other 120 milligrams of ginkgo twice a day, beginning five days before ascent. All of the volunteers were then taken rapidly to a very high altitude (14,100 feet), where they spent the night. Those taking the ginkgo experienced about 50 percent fewer episodes of acute mountain sickness compared to the placebo group, and those who did become ill had fewer and milder symptoms than the control group. The report, presented at the Wilderness Medical Society 2000 summer conference, concluded that 120 milligrams of ginkgo, taken twice a day beginning five days before going to a higher altitude and continuing during any additional ascent, was effective in preventing AMS.

SUMMING UP

Most heart patients can travel safely, but preventive measures may be needed. Talk to your doctor before flying or embarking on a trip: doing so not only will help ease any worries but also can prevent complications.

IV

Advances
in Treating
Heart Disease
and Hope
for the Future

Heretofore, we have concentrated on the two key components of treating cardiovascular disease: namely, the importance of understanding the nature of your individual disease and the need to commit to a life-long plan designed to provide the best outcomes. This commitment requires that you, as a patient, become an integral member of your health management team. It involves both lifestyle changes and when appropriate, medical therapy. It requires not only learning about your condition, but also working with your doctor to modify or effectively treat it. But the educational process does not stop with today's approaches. Just as the disease may change over time, so too have treatment options evolved. To be the most effective partner in your own care, you should be aware of ongoing research that will ultimately bring increased understanding of, and new means of managing, cardiovascular disease.

The media have helped increase public awareness of new advances. But the media focus is all too often fleeting, sensationalized, and incomplete or even distorted. These reports often lack comprehensible explanations of the underlying science on the assumption that the general public either isn't interested or lacks the background to understand technical concepts. So today's headlines or sound bites are quickly forgotten as "old news."

Such fleeting attention is unfortunate because an understanding of research trends and new treatments will help you learn how you may benefit from them. Such knowledge also provides hope, as you rationally study your disease and make a treatment plan. Hope in this sense is a way of directing your natural fear of the unknown away from despair, yet involves far more than blind, wishful thinking. As stated eloquently by Dr. Jerome Groopman in his book *Anatomy of Hope:* "Hope incorporates fear into the process of rational deliberation and tempers it so we can think and choose without panic."

Hope should be an important component of every patient's attitude. This is not mere witchcraft or psychobabble. Research focusing on the brain-body interaction has frequently shown substantial and direct links among how we think, our emotions, our approaches to stress, and a multitude of complex clinical and physiological events. These medical responses range from the chest pains of angina pectoris, heart attacks, and sudden cardiac death, to immunologic resistance, gastrointestinal disease, and even alteration of the structure and perhaps function of chromosomes, the fundamental carriers of genetic information.

Nowhere is there a greater reason for hope of improved human health than in the area of cardiovascular disease. No other field of medicine has demonstrated such sustained and well-documented evidence of improvement in the survival and well-being of patients. These remarkable strides can be attributed both to major changes in patients' lifestyles as well as to the development and establishment of multiple new therapeutic strategies. Over the almost forty years since I graduated from medical school, extraordinary advances have dramatically changed heart care, and halved the death toll from cardiovascular disease. These changes, which typically begin in the research laboratory, are ultimately incorporated into direct patient care.

This part addresses exciting new clinical trials and potential advances in cardiovascular care. Some of these advances are already being adopted into patient care, others are entering into clinical research trials involving patients, and still others are being tested in experimental animals. Although they may not all live up to their initial promise, it is clear that within the next decade new therapies, based on a deeper understanding of the biology of heart disease, will emerge from the experimental arena—and become available to your physician and you as you work together to help manage or cure your disease.

15

Recently Developed
Devices and Procedures

In recent decades, the treatment of cardiovascular disease has been revolutionized by the development of highly effective medications and exciting new procedures and operative techniques. Many of these treatments are now becoming routine in modern cardiovascular care, but they are only part of an ongoing process. New devices and procedures, as well as medications, are being introduced at an amazing pace, and even more are being developed and tested in laboratories and research centers throughout the United States and abroad. In this chapter, we offer a brief overview of some of the new devices and procedures. Given the scope and purpose of this book, we make no attempt to be all-inclusive; instead, we concentrate on those that have already generated significant interest within medical and research circles. Of course, this does not mean that all will live up to their initial promise, and what's new and exciting today may well be rendered obsolete tomorrow by either new research or even more refined developments. Still, it's important for you, as a lay reader and present or possible future heart patient, to be aware of these new developments. As you develop your own long-term treatment plan, knowledge of likely future advances is not only a source of hope, but can also become part of your plan for the future.

SURGICAL PROCEDURES

Over the last forty years, cardiovascular surgery has undergone incredible advances, beginning with the introduction of the heart-lung machine in the 1960s to provide circulation during open-heart surgery. Open-heart operations involve opening the chest cavity and stopping the heart to enable surgeons to bypass clogged coronary arteries, repair or replace defective valves, and carry out other procedures. While open-heart surgery in itself is amazing, it is now as well possible to perform surgery without using the heart-lung machine (that is, "off pump") and by "keyhole" procedures that allow surgeons to operate on a beating heart through a small incision. Even more astonishing surgical procedures either are becoming available or are in the final stages of development.

Surgical Ventricular Restoration

Surgery to treat advanced coronary artery disease often involves operating on patients who already have had major heart attacks (myocardial infarctions, or MIs). At times, the parts of the heart that have sustained major damage become thin-walled and bulging; when this occurs in the heart's main pumping chamber, it is called a left ventricular aneurysm. The scarred and weakened heart muscle in these areas reduces overall heart function and can lead to heart failure.

We have learned from numerous animal experiments and human autopsy studies that a heart attack causes the most havoc to the inner portion of the heart muscle wall. The outer margin of the heart muscle, even in the area of the heart attack, is often preserved. Yet surgeons seeking to improve heart function for heart-attack patients have for years resorted to a procedure called an aneurysm resection (aneurysmectomy), in which the entire area, including normal tissue, is removed.

New surgical techniques now under development and testing involve removing mostly the inner portion of the heart wall that has been most damaged by the heart attack while leaving the outer portion intact. The surgical repair involves using a part of the actual scar tissue from the heart attack as a patch to reduce the tension on the wall of the heart and help prevent further expansion of the heart muscle. This approach not only results in a more normal shape of the left ventricle, but also helps prevent some of the untoward effects of remodeling the chamber. The heart size is reduced and the function of the area in the heart unaffected by the heart attack is improved.

A number of published studies describing the technique have detailed the initial promising results. As of this writing, at least one large-scale study is under way to evaluate further how successful this surgical treatment is in relation to other medical and surgical therapies.

Left Ventricular Assist Devices/Artificial Heart

Although significant strides have been made in the medical treatment of patients with heart failure, this form of cardiovascular disease remains a leading cause of cardiac death. For a long time, a heart transplant using a donor organ was the only major surgical treatment available for advanced heart failure. But the shortage of suitable donor organs greatly limits this transplantation as a widespread treatment of this condition.

Beginning in the 1960s, mechanical devices to bolster the heart's pumping ability have been used, and these continue to evolve. The early mechanical assistance devices included short-term use of a balloon pump placed in the patient's aorta to boost the heart's pumping function. Over time, more long-lasting devices have been introduced, with the ultimate goal of developing a completely artificial heart that can be used until a donor heart becomes available. To date, models of experimental artificial hearts have been used in a few instances, with the promise of less cumbersome and more effective models to come.

Considerable success has been achieved with ventricular assist devices (VADs). Developed initially as temporary aids for patients with very advanced heart failure who were waiting for a donor heart, these devices are now considered an ultimate or "destination therapy." Studies are now under way to define the indications for VAD implantation to better identify patients most likely to benefit from it. At present, a number of different VADs are either available or being tested. These vary according to size, surgical procedure required to implant them, the type of blood flow they produce, and the connections required within the chest. Although all VADs require implantation, the nature of the operation varies. For example, some devices are totally implantable, while others may have external controls.

Already these devices are having a significant effect on patient care. A recent study demonstrated their benefits in comparison to conventional medical therapy, despite the risk of complications such as bleeding, infection, blood clots, mechanical failure of the devices, and failure of the right side of the heart. Because of such serious complications, this new and rather aggressive treatment is being reserved for extremely ill patients. As the devices are further refined, however, VAD implantation holds considerable promise as a therapy for other patients as well.

Robotic Surgery

Heart surgery traditionally has involved placing patients on a heart-lung machine and opening the chest to expose the heart and other organs. As less-invasive techniques requiring relatively small incisions become more common, however, robotic telemanipulation systems—in which an operation can be directed by a surgeon at a distant location—may become increasingly commonplace.

There are generally two types of robotic surgery: In one system, the robotic device functions as a tool that the on-site surgical team can use to hold and position surgical instruments during the operation. The robot, for example, can be programmed to hold a specific position or to move to a different one.

A second type of robotic system is designed to help with fine manipulations that are done at a remote site. The robotic device is controlled by an operator who works at a special console, allowing for very precise surgical manipulation in very small spaces. Although this sounds like something out of *Star Wars* or some other sci-fi drama, in practice the robot is exquisitely stable and does not allow any movements that have not been carefully programmed.

These techniques are currently done predominately for valve surgery, particularly repair of the mitral valve. But it is possible or even likely that this exciting new approach will expand to broader heart surgery applications. It is likely that the devices will become even smaller, and as surgeons develop greater experience and facility, robotic heart surgery may become more frequently and routinely performed.

Transmyocardial Laser Revascularization

Transmyocardial laser revascularization, which has received considerable media attention in the past few years, involves using a laser during surgery to create small new channels within the heart muscle wall. The goal is to improve blood flow to areas of the heart that are not amenable to more conventional approaches such as bypass surgery. Although initial results appeared promising, other well-controlled studies have failed to substantiate them; consequently, it appears that this technique is unlikely to be used alone to improve blood flow to the heart. But it may have a future role as a way during bypass surgery to provide improved blood flow to certain areas that would not be helped by more conventional forms of revascularization. In addition, this technique might be useful for delivering other biologically active treatments to diseased tissue. (See Chapter 16.)

CARDIOLOGY PROCEDURES

Just as in the case of surgery, major advances have occurred in cardiology procedures. Some of these procedures are done in the cardiac catheterization laboratory; others are done in a more specialized catheterization laboratory and cover an area called electrophysiology. In general, these procedures are performed by cardiologists who have additional training.

Angioplasty and Related Procedures

These procedures, referred to as percutaneous coronary intervention or PCI, include balloon angioplasty of the coronary arteries, which was first performed in 1977. Initially, balloon angioplasty was limited to patients with disease of the first portion of one coronary artery. As the field has evolved and equipment has improved, the uses of angioplasty have expanded to include the assistance of patients with disease in multiple coronary arteries and the treatment of more complex blockages.

Over the last decade, additional devices have been developed to improve results. One of the most important of these was the development of coronary stents, tiny devices that are inserted into the arteries to keep the treated arteries open. Stents are now used in the overwhelming majority of angioplasty procedures. Other major advances in percutaneous intervention include:

Drug-Eluting Stents

Heretofore, a major problem in the use of coronary stents involved a subsequent narrowing at the site of placement. This generally occurs because of an overgrowth of cells (hyperplasia) within the wall of the blood vessel, resulting in a narrowing referred to as restenosis. The likelihood of restenosis is reduced to less than 10 percent by using new drug-eluting stents, which contain chemicals in their walls that prevent cell growth in the adjacent vessel wall. These new stents are positioned and placed in much the same manner as their earlier counterparts and they do not appear to increase the risk of adverse effects. They also appear to be equally effective in men and women. (For more on stents, see Figure 10 in Chapter 7.)

Brachytherapy

Used primarily to treat stent restenosis, brachytherapy involves the direct delivery of radiation through the catheter tip to destroy a small amount of tissue at the site of restenosis. Although this technique has been quite effective in preventing restenosis, it is likely to be used less frequently as the use of drug-eluting stents becomes more widespread.

Coronary Atherectomy

Coronary atherectomy was developed in the early 1990s. Performed during angioplasty, it involves removing part of the fatty deposits in the coronary artery (atherosclerotic plaque). In traditional balloon angioplasty, the plaque is flattened when the balloon is inflated; in contrast, during atherectomy the plaque is cut away and removed. The devices used are called either directional or rotational, referring to the manner in which the plaque is removed. Atherectomy generally results in a wider artery channel than can be achieved with a balloon alone. Although atherectomy has been somewhat replaced by stenting and other newer techniques, it still fills a specific need.

Distal Embolic Protection Devices

A possible complication of angioplasty occurs when debris from the atherosclerotic plaque breaks away from the artery wall and moves downstream in the artery being treated, possibly resulting in blockage of small downstream blood vessels. This complication is most common when large plaques develop in a venous coronary bypass graft. To help prevent it, special catheters have been developed that contain downstream filters to prevent debris from passing into the coronary circulation. When the filters are removed at the end of the procedure, any debris that has been captured in them is also removed.

Angioplasty in Other Obstructed Vessels

The angioplasty techniques used to treat coronary artery disease can be used in other blood vessels. For example, we now have extensive experience in using angioplasty to treat blocked blood vessels in the legs, kidneys, and the carotid arteries in the neck, which supply blood to the brain. Angioplasty on the carotid arteries usually includes techniques performed with filters to prevent bits of plaque from reaching the brain and causing a stroke (see earlier). It is expected that angioplasty will become the predominant therapy for occluded blood vessels in other parts of the body, and in some instances, may replace or diminish the current surgical techniques used to open narrowed arteries.

Intravascular Therapy of Aortic Aneurysms

Techniques are being developed to allow percutaneous placement of stent-grafts into the aorta, the body's largest artery that arises from the heart and supplies blood to the arterial system. An aortic aneurysm involves an outward bulging at a weakened segment of the artery; this commonly develops in the abdominal aorta and can be life-threatening if it ruptures. Treatment with stent-grafts is still under development, but initial results have been promising. If successful, this approach can eliminate the need for major surgery to repair the aneurysm.

Patent Foramen Ovale and Atrial Septal Defect Closure

A patent foramen ovale (PFO) is a persistent flap-like opening between the two atria (upper chambers of the heart). This condition can lead to a stroke, particularly in young individuals. The cause of the stroke is presumably a small blood clot that passes from the veins of the lower extremities into the right heart and then across this opening and into the blood circulation to the brain. When treatment with anticoagulation drugs is not effective, the PFO can be closed directly with an occluding device that is put in place during cardiac catheterization. The same approach can be used to close larger atrial septal defects—congenital openings in the wall between the two atria—thereby avoiding the need for heart surgery.

Treatment of Heart-Valve Disorders

Endovascular treatment of heart-valve disorders in the cardiac catheterization laboratory is not widely used and has not been nearly as effective as when used to treat narrowed coronary arteries and other blood vessels. There are, however, circumstances in which it is beneficial. These include widening with balloon techniques a narrowed mitral valve (percutaneous mitral balloon valvotomy), pulmonic valve in children or young adults, or aortic valve—although in the case of the aortic valve the treatment is not as beneficial and generally is reserved for conditions in which aortic valve surgery would be extremely hazardous. Because these techniques are not widely used, if they are to be undertaken, they should be done only in institutions where a significant number of these procedures have been performed.

Another approach, which is still experimental and in the very early stages of development, involves replacement of defective valves using percutaneous techniques. This valve-replacement therapy has already been performed successfully in several patients. If the technique proves to be effective, it would represent a major advance in interventional cardiology, and replace some of the more invasive surgical techniques that are now widely used.

Septal Ablation for Hypertrophic Cardiomyopathy

Hypertrophic cardiomyopathy is a form of heart muscle disease (cardiomyopathy) that involves the overgrowth (hypertrophy) of heart muscle tissue. One form of hypertrophic cardiomyopathy involves asymmetrical thickening of the wall (septum) that separates the left and right ventricles—the lower chambers of the heart. The condition can impede the flow of blood that is being pumped from the left ventricle into the aorta. Also known as idiopathic hypertropic subaortic stenosis, or IHSS, it is the most common cause of sudden death in young athletes in the United States. It can often be treated with medication, but severe cases may require surgical removal of a portion of the thickened septum. Recently, techniques have been developed whereby alcohol is infused into the artery supplying blood to the septum, causing the destruction and thinning of a portion of the septal wall. This procedure can reduce symptoms and may reduce possible complications of the condition.

Enhanced External Counterpulsation

Although most patients with coronary artery disease and angina pectoris can be treated with medication, bypass surgery, or the interventional cardiology techniques described earlier, new strategies are being considered to help the small but significant number of patients for whom these approaches do not work or cannot be used. One such strategy is enhanced external counterpulsation (EECP), a novel technique that has been evaluated in several large studies. The technique, which involves thirty-five one-hour therapy sessions over four to seven weeks, can be performed in an office or outpatient setting. During the session, three sets of cuffs are wrapped around each leg, at the lower leg and lower and upper thigh. These cuffs are attached to a device that allows the expansion of the cuffs to be synchronized with each heartbeat. The cuffs expand under pressure sequentially from the lower to upper portions of the lower extremity. This propels blood back to the heart from the veins in the legs. Rapid deflation of the cuffs lowers the resistance against which the heart must pump.

This technique appears to be the most beneficial for patients who suffer from severe angina and are not candidates for more conventional treatments. Those who have undergone EECP report fewer episodes of angina and increased ability to exercise. How the technique produces these positive results is not fully understood, but several possible explanations have been put forth. These include direct effects on circulation, the development of collateral blood vessels within the heart, and production of substances within the body that improve vessel function and blood flow.

Ablation for Cardiac Arrhythmias

A number of medications, many of them listed in Chapter 7, have been developed to treat a variety of supraventricular cardiac arrhythmias. In a number of instances, however, these medications are not effective. Consequently, a technique called catheter ablation, which is carried out in an electrophysiology laboratory, has been developed. Ablation is designed to eliminate the site where these rhythm disturbances arise by destroying a small, well-defined area of heart tissue. The ablation entails delivering electrical energy through a catheter, which is placed in the precise part of the heart that has been determined to be causing the trouble. The energy destroys the small area of heart tissue responsible for the arrhythmia by controlled heat production at the site of the catheter tip. The treatment is the most effective in eliminating rapid heart rhythms that originate in the upper portion (supraventricular area) of the heart. The technique requires precise localization of the source of rhythm disturbance in the electrophysiology laboratory before the delivery of the energy. Although the procedure is highly sophisticated, it is now available nationwide. Clearly, the elimination of a heart rhythm disturbance through a single, generally safe procedure has many advantages over taking medication for recurring episodes of supraventricular tachycardia.

Other, perhaps more complicated, ablation techniques are being developed to treat atrial flutter and atrial fibrillation—abnormal rhythms affecting the upper chambers of the heart. Although ablation techniques for atrial fibrillation are still evolving, a number of different approaches are under study and show promise in eliminating this very common rhythm disturbance, which also carries an increased risk of a stroke.

Cardiac Resynchronization Therapy

One of the more exciting developments in the treatment of heart failure involves the use of biventricular pacing in selected patients to improve heart function and reduce symptoms. Pacemakers have been employed for decades to treat heart block—when the atria and ventricles beat in an uncoordinated way—or extremely slow heart rates. These pacemakers have become highly sophisticated in how they sense problems and deliver their stimuli; they also have become miniaturized. But there is now awareness that certain patients, specifically those with ventricular conduction delay, may benefit from ensuring that the two ventricles of the heart beat in a synchronized fashion. This is done with biventricular pacing.

Studies of cardiac resynchronization therapy, or CRT, have shown that the treatment can potentially improve symptoms and lead to longer survival in at least 15 to 30 percent of patients with advanced heart failure. The technique, which is highly complex, involves placing catheters in both ventricles to ensure a smooth and synchronous contraction within the heart. Newer devices combine this pacemaker with a defibrillator (see later in this chapter).

Implantable Cardioverter-Defibrillator

Implantable cardioverter-defibrillators (ICDs) are small devices placed in and near the heart. They are designed to deliver an electrical shock within the heart to convert a potentially lethal rhythm disturbance to a normal heart rhythm. Numerous studies have established the efficacy of ICDs, which are now routinely implanted in individuals who have survived a cardiac arrest or are at high risk of life-threatening arrhythmias, usually ventricular tachycardia. Candidates for ICDs include patients with serious coronary artery disease and a history of heart attacks and depressed heart function. Ventricular tachycardia may also occur in patients who have heart muscle disease (cardiomyopathy) or some relatively unusual forms of inherited heart disease such as Brugada syndrome or Long QT syndrome. (See Chapters 7 and 12.)

It is now clear that ICDs have even wider applications. For example, there is benefit in implanting ICDs in patients who have seriously depressed heart function (for example, when the left ventricle pumps out less than 30 percent of the blood in its chamber with each heartbeat). These low ejection fractions may occur following heart attacks or in patients with cardiomyopathy. In these patients, an ICD may be implanted even if there is no known cardiac arrhythmia, and studies have demonstrated significant improvement in their survival. Consequently, ICDs are now recommended in such individuals—yet another major advance in our understanding and treatment of heart disease.

SUMMING UP

The development of new devices and procedures is a fertile and expanding area. These new advances can have a positive effect on many aspects of heart disease, thereby significantly improving symptoms and survival rates. Indeed, there is every reason to assume that devices and procedures will continue to evolve and improve, providing ever more sophisticated and beneficial care for those patients who may need it.

16

Biologically Based Therapies

The revolution in molecular and cell biology has led to a remarkable understanding of the biology of the cardiovascular system. This new knowledge has also been applied to developing entirely new forms of treatment. In this chapter we will briefly review three types of such biologically based therapies: growing new blood vessels, stem cell therapy, and gene therapy. Research advances in those areas are among the most exciting new approaches to the treatment of cardiovascular disease, although each has possible drawbacks.

GROWING NEW BLOOD VESSELS

At present, persons who suffer from serious heart disease, such as frequent bouts of chest pain due to angina pectoris (myocardial ischemia), or those who have had a heart attack (myocardial infarction, or MI), are treated with either medications or invasive procedures, such as angioplasty or coronary artery bypass graft surgery (CABG). These treatments, discussed in detail in Chapters 7 and 15, are intended to relieve symptoms by increasing blood flow to the heart muscle. Yet although most patients benefit from these treatments, there are those who don't receive adequate relief. For example, some patients are not good candidates for angioplasty or CABG because their coronary arteries are too small, or the buildup of fatty deposits (atherosclerosis) is too extensive. For some of these patients, even the most aggressive drug therapy does not provide enough improvement. In such circumstances, the ability to stimulate growth of new blood vessels—a process called neovascularization—within the heart would provide a major therapeutic advance. In addition, stimulation of new blood vessel growth early after a heart attack could prevent certain complications, such as the type of enlargement we refer to as cardiac restructuring or "remodeling," that can lead ultimately to heart failure. In some instances, then, new blood vessel growth could be an effective treatment for certain types of heart failure.

Just a few years ago, the idea of growing new blood vessels was considered futuristic speculation. But over the past decade, new advances in blood vessel biology have demonstrated that new growth may soon become a reality. There are three types of new blood vessel development. The first, vasculogenesis, involves the formation of entirely new blood vessels from progenitor cells. This process occurs naturally in the developing embryo, but not much thereafter; the idea is to "turn on" this process again for therapeutic purposes. Angiogenesis, another approach, involves the formation of new capillaries (very small blood vessels) from existing blood vessels. And in arteriogenesis, newly formed or existing channels are remodeled into large, well-muscularized blood vessels to form arterioles and additional new collateral blood vessels.

These revascularization processes are stimulated by a number of factors and involve a complex interaction of new cell division (proliferation) and formation of these newly formed cells into specific cell types suitable for forming blood vessels (differentiation). Within the body, this process is stimulated by inadequate levels of oxygen in the tissue (hypoxia) as well as inflammation and additional physical forces (shear stress) placed on the heart muscle. Other circulating chemicals in the blood, such as growth factors, also play a significant role. The complex interaction between the presence and activity of these growth factors and timing can stimulate the local area to stabilize and lead to maturation of the new blood vessels. (See Figure 11.)

Role of Growth Factors

Vascular growth factors play an extremely important role in the overall process of forming new blood vessels. In recent years, an increased understanding of this biology has led to the actual therapeutic use of growth factors to stimulate new blood vessel development. There are a number of different but interrelated families of growth factors that stimulate new vessel development. They also increase

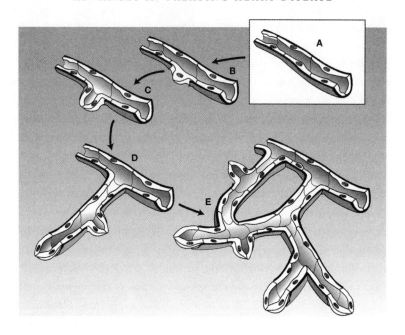

FIGURE 11. How new blood vessels grow when stimulated. Growth factors stimulate development of new blood vessels from the original vessel (A) to increase the delivery of blood to the adjacent areas (B through E).

the presence of cells from the bone marrow, known as endothelial progenitor cells, that can stimulate this process. A significant number of studies using experimental animals have shown positive results with these forms of therapy.

Several clinical trials, involving modest numbers of patients, are under way. These are aimed at demonstrating the effectiveness of employing various growth factors in humans to stimulate the growth of new blood vessels. These trials have involved vascular endothelial growth factor (VEGF) as well as fibroblast growth factor (FGF), which can be injected directly into the coronary artery during angiography or injected into the heart muscle during cardiac surgery. Both growth factors, as well as the genes leading to growth factor production, have been employed. To date, these studies have yielded somewhat complex, and, at times, conflicting results. The potential of this approach has continued to stimulate major research, even though the field has not established clear-cut benefits and there are many questions that still need to be answered. For example, should growth factors be administered into the coronary artery, intravenously, or into the heart muscle directly? Should the growth factor be administered as a protein or in the form of its actual gene?

In addition, there are several at least theoretical issues that must be addressed before the technique is ready for widespread clinical use. Will it result in excessive or otherwise unwanted blood vessel growth? Such a side effect could be potentially harmful if it occurs in the retina of the eye of a particularly vulnerable person, such as someone with diabetes. Does the new blood vessel function in an entirely normal manner or does it allow material to pass through its walls because of increased permeability? In addition, it is known that increased blood vessel growth is key to the spread of cancer, so is this a potential hazard for persons who may harbor unrecognized tumors?

Other New Approaches

Another new approach to stimulating blood vessel growth involves the direct administration of endothelial progenitor cells (EPC) from the patient's bone marrow or circulation. Small numbers of these cells circulate in the blood normally and are produced within the bone marrow. Normally these cells repair injured blood vessels that may occur in response to a number of circumstances.

Several studies have demonstrated that the collection and harvesting of these endothelial progenitor cells can be used to stimulate new blood vessel growth when administered to either experimental animals or patients. Consequently, this approach can provide an entirely new means for inducing the growth of new blood vessels, or vasculogenesis. There are also apparent interactions between enhanced endothelial progenitor cell circulation and the presence of cytokines— a type of protein that acts as a cellular mediator—or growth factors such as VEGF. In addition, recent studies have shown that the drugs used for cholesterol lowering (the statins) augment the mobilization of endothelial progenitor cells from the bone marrow.

Much research is still needed in the area of building new blood vessels. But results to date justify considerable excitement and optimism. Future work will involve defining the optimal means of inducing new blood vessel growth, as well as the best way to administer the new treatments, which will probably involve combined therapy with both growth factors and endothelial progenitor cells. It also seems likely that many other groups of patients, not just those for whom there are no other options, but also those undergoing treatment of a heart attack and other heart problems, will benefit from this approach—and that it can also be employed to help generate blood vessels in areas other than the heart, such as other organs or the legs.

THE POTENTIAL OF STEM CELLS IN CARDIOLOGY

Every cell, tissue, and organ in the body starts from stem cells. These are undifferentiated or "blank" cells that the body can program to carry out the functions of any of the body's tissues or organs; they also are unique because they can make many copies of themselves before dying. These stem cells have become the focus of intense scientific interest and political discord. Because of their singular properties, they are a promising source of cells to treat any number of debilitating and fatal diseases, ranging from spinal cord injuries and Parkinson's disease to heart failure and other forms of cardiovascular disease. In a future field that is referred to as regenerative medicine, stem cells could potentially be used to create healthy organs or tissue to replace the body's diseased ones.

Sources of Stem Cells

Controversy and ethical questions arise over the source of stem cells. Let's begin with a very brief overview of human biology. All life starts with a single cell, called a zygote, which is formed from an egg (ovum) that has been fertilized by a sperm, the male reproductive cell. Within hours of fertilization, the zygote begins to divide, forming two, then four, then eight cells and so forth until after about five days the zygote becomes a blastocyst, a hollow cluster—smaller than a grain of sand—that is made up of about 150 cells. The inner cells are called embryonic or pluripotent stem cells, and it is these cells that ultimately form all the cell types in a living human being.

Fetal stem cells, which are similar to their embryonic counterparts, are found in the blood of a newborn's umbilical cord. Scientists have also discovered stem cells in baby teeth and the amniotic fluid, the liquid that surrounds the fetus in the uterus.

In addition to embryonic and fetal stem cells, a small number of stem cells exist in the adult body, especially in the bone marrow and, to a lesser degree, the brain and perhaps other organs. These adult multipotent stem cells or progenitor cells can form cell types of multiple organs. Thus, stem cells from the bone marrow give rise to all types of blood cells. As more is learned about how these bone-marrow-derived cells function, scientists are hopeful that these adult stem cells can be stimulated to produce a wider range of tissues, and thus be used to regenerate diseased organs and cure disorders that are untreatable or treatable only by organ transplantation. Indeed, stem cells may currently offer the greatest opportunity for regeneration in the heart.

After stem cells have been isolated, they can be grown for long periods of time—perhaps even indefinitely—in a laboratory setting. The cells are placed in special incubators that contain growth factors and are exposed to temperatures and mixtures of oxygen and carbon dioxide that mimic conditions inside the human body. When removed from these incubators and exposed to the right stimuli, the stem cells can be programmed to form specific tissues or organs.

Ethical issues have arisen over the creation and use of embryonic stem cells. At present, most embryonic stem cells come from the excess embryos created in fertility clinics. Opponents to stem cell research and use argue that it is unethical to destroy a potential life to treat an existing person. Supporters counter that the embryos would be destroyed in any event, and that it is ethical to use them to further science and benefit sick or dying humans. These ethical issues are beyond the scope of this chapter; instead, what follows concentrates on the potential of using stem cells to treat some forms of cardiovascular disease.

Treating Heart Failure with Stem Cells

The development of congestive heart failure remains a major problem in cardiovascular disease. This condition is most often caused by repeated heart attacks and loss of heart muscle tissue. As more and more heart muscle is lost, the main pumping chamber—the left ventricle—begins to enlarge, changing its shape and ultimately, its function. This process is called ventricular remodeling. While current therapies using medication, heart surgery, or cardiac interventional procedures have certainly been of great benefit, heart failure remains a serious problem, resulting in the largest number of hospital admissions for cardiovascular disease in the United States.

Research has demonstrated that within the heart muscle itself there exists the potential for regeneration or development of new muscle cells. This is a new and somewhat revolutionary concept, since previously it was believed that heart muscle cells were incapable of regeneration following their injury or death. Growing evidence also has been obtained in both experimental animals and humans indicating that delivery of stem cells to areas of heart muscle injury can result in a repopulation of normal cells in the damaged area with ultimate improvement in cardiac function.

A variety of stem cells have been used to accomplish this regeneration.

These relatively primitive cells have an enormous potential for differentiation—specifically, transforming themselves into the cells of a specific organ cell type. Some of the initial studies have used endothelial progenitor cells, which are derived from the bone marrow but also circulate in small numbers in the bloodstream. These have the potential of forming new blood vessels and other cells in the heart. Other studies have employed actual smooth muscle cells, embryonic stem cells, and/or fetal myocytes, which are cells taken from fetal skeletal muscle and subsequently placed in the heart. Stem cells derived from bone marrow, circulating blood, or skeletal muscle all can be obtained from the individual patient who subsequently will then receive them, thus sidestepping the issue of obtaining stem cells from fetuses or embryos. In the clinical research arena of cardiac regeneration, adult bone marrow stem cells, derived from the patient to whom they will be administered, have been used most often. It also should be noted that stem cells derived from other tissues, such as fat tissue or umbilical cord blood, contain a large number of endogenous embryonic stem cells that could be saved for future use.

Does This Technique Work?

Experimental studies to date have provided some impressive results. For example, remarkable improvement has been demonstrated in experimental animals following the delivery of stem cells to the areas in need of repair. It is likely that once these cells take hold in the heart muscle they actually differentiate and repopulate the areas rather than fusing directly with already damaged cells.

Experimental studies have advanced from mice to humans, and several initial preliminary reports have demonstrated both safety and apparent efficacy. The human studies, however, have involved relatively small numbers of patients and have not been rigorously controlled. They have also not been without controversy. Clearly, before the use of stem cells to regenerate heart tissue can become more widespread, larger clinical research trials are needed. (See Figure 12 for an overview of the proposed procedure.)

Challenges to Overcome

As might be expected, many questions remain. For example, what is the best way of delivering these stem cells to the heart muscle? Much research still needs to be done to determine the actual homing signals that direct these stem cells to the

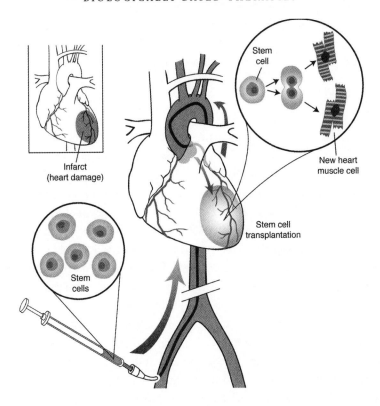

FIGURE 12. Using stem cells to grow new heart muscle. After a heart attack, part of the damaged heart muscle dies (insert at upper left). As part of an experiment, stem cells have been injected via a coronary catheter into such areas, where they have developed into new heart muscle and blood vessel cells. Although more research is needed, initial results are promising.

appropriate area. Understanding this basic mechanism may allow for the development of additional and more simple means of delivering stem cells.

Currently, a number of sophisticated approaches are being used to deliver stem cells to their target organs. These include direct surgical implantation; delivery into the coronary artery through a catheter similar to those employed for routine angiography or interventional cardiology; and other more complex catheter techniques that involve mapping the inner lining of the left ventricle to determine optimal site for delivery and then directing delivery through the catheter into the area most suitable for repair. Perhaps in the future, the homing process will become understood to the extent that a patient could receive an intravenous injection of cells and they would go right to where they are needed; to date, we don't know how to accomplish this goal.

Remaining Questions

Although many technical questions remain to be answered, none are unduly daunting or markedly different from those that face any revolutionary new therapy. These questions include: How do we identify the patients who would be the best candidates for stem cell therapy? When is the optimal time for delivering stem cells following a heart attack? Can this therapy be employed in patients who have not had a recent heart attack, but nevertheless have older heart damage? If the cells are administered early during a heart attack, would they be destroyed along with the existing cardiac cells? To date, the best experimental results have occurred shortly after a heart attack. Will the same hold true when the damaged heart tissue has been replaced by scar tissue?

There are also questions as to which stem cells are the most effective. A variety of stem cells have been employed in initial studies, but we still do not know which type produces the best results. Also, very little is known about how these stem cells ultimately achieve success. By what mechanisms do these cells home in on a specific area, settle there, and then ultimately differentiate into new heart cells? How long do these cells live once present in the heart? Is there uniform improvement in heart function following this therapy? Will the therapy be associated with long-term risks, such as heart rhythm disorders or tumor formation?

Despite these remaining questions and potential problems, stem cells constitute a most exciting potential new approach for treating serious heart disease. It is not unreasonable to consider a future in which progenitor cells from patients' own bone marrow will be combined with other forms of pharmacologic therapy, interventional cardiology, surgery, or even gene therapy to restore the previously damaged heart. Perhaps one day we will even be able to harness the amazing therapeutic potential of progenitor cells to slow or in some ways reverse human aging.

GENE THERAPY

Gene therapy is yet another biologically based, and promising, potential way of treating or preventing cardiovascular disease. Despite reports of complications in a few patients undergoing experimental gene therapy for disorders outside the cardiovascular system, the technique nevertheless offers reason for cautious optimism.

Gene therapy can be defined as the introduction of new genetic material into a cell or tissue to produce a new pattern of genetic expression. In this setting, the therapy comes from a protein expressed by the new gene. Suppose, for example, that the heart lacks a specific protein that could protect against a heart attack. Conceivably, the introduction of genetic material that can cause production of the protein could prompt the heart to replenish this protein, thereby helping to prevent the possibility of heart attack in the patient. Similar genetic approaches can be applied to other organ systems and diseases.

There are several steps in this process. First, the gene of interest must be identified among the many thousands of possible candidate genes. It then must be characterized chemically and reproduced through cloning techniques. Next, the cloned DNA for the gene is linked to a carrier—called a vector—that helps introduce the genetic material into the target tissue. This foreign genetic material then enters the nucleus of the cells and ultimately becomes incorporated into its genetic structure, thereby leading to the expression of the desired missing protein.

While this may sound relatively straightforward, in reality it is an extremely complex process. Despite the extensive genetic research that has already been done, many questions remain unanswered. Although excellent results have been obtained in animal models of disease, human studies have been somewhat limited and there have been a few instances of negative results, including at least one patient death.

Areas of Potential Benefit

In addition to promoting growth of new blood vessels, there are a number of other cardiovascular targets in which gene therapy could prove beneficial. These include excessive growth of muscle tissue in arteries, particularly after angioplasty; clot development (thrombosis); cell death; and instability of fatty deposits in blood vessels (atherosclerotic plaque). Recent studies in experimental animals indicate that gene therapy may reduce tissue injury after a heart attack or prolonged lack of oxygen (ischemia or oxidative stress). Gene therapy has also been shown to protect coronary artery bypasses made from a portion of saphenous vein taken from the leg. It may also protect against inflammation, a common cause of tissue damage.

Still, a number of questions require detailed study. A major issue involves identifying the ideal vector to carry the genetic material to the target site(s). In many instances an altered virus is used as a vector, but it is not known whether the virus may produce its own negative effects. Other questions center around delivery techniques, which currently include injections into the coronary arteries or direct injection into heart muscle. Safety, too, is a concern, given that in an early U.S. gene therapy trial an eighteen-year-old male patient unexpectedly died, and in a French study involving immunologically compromised children, several have developed leukemia following gene therapy. It is also unclear at this point how best to determine the success of gene therapy. Clearly, long-term follow-up of patients will be a critical part of this effort.

As more is learned about the biology of cardiovascular disease, we can expect refined techniques and increased targets for gene therapy. Although caution is needed, gene therapy represents yet another area of optimism for the future.

SUMMING UP

To a greater extent than ever before, extraordinary advances in modern basic science are being harnessed to create new treatments for cardiovascular disease. The exciting research in new blood vessel development, stem cell therapy, and gene therapy is likely only the beginning. Work in these areas will expand and develop, while new areas of potential treatment involving biologically based therapies will appear on the scene. Clearly, there is substantial scientific reason for patients and their families to feel hopeful that they, too, will benefit from these discoveries and their applications to heart disease.

17

Experimental Treatments
and Clinical Trials

C linical trials—scientific studies that involve human subjects—are the method by which new medical treatments are evaluated for safety and effectiveness. At one time, the general public was barely aware of this process; in recent years, however, the results of clinical trials have made headlines, often prematurely. These days, the public often learns the results of important clinical trials when a company, agency, or sometimes the researchers themselves hold a press conference or issue a press release, often at the time of initial presentation at a professional society. Almost immediately the media report the "news," often with great fanfare or hype that may go beyond the actual relevance of the study itself. Patients start calling their doctors for information on the new "breakthrough," often before it has been evaluated scientifically or approved for general use. Thus, it's important to understand the nature of clinical trials, so that you can both assess possibly premature or misleading media reports and decide whether you want to try to participate in a study involving experimental medications or treatments (see Table 18 for an illustrative list of clinical trials).

WHO PERFORMS CLINICAL TRIALS?

Clinical trials often take place in hospitals and major academic medical centers, or in physician offices. They are most often sponsored and supported by the

TABLE 18

EXAMPLES OF CLINICAL TRIALS PRESENTED IN 2004–2005

Trial	Number of Patients Involved	Major Question of Study
TNT (Treating to New Targets)	10,001	Does lowering LDL cholesterol to less than usual therapeutic levels provide additional benefit?
ASCOT (Anglo-Scandinavian Cardiac Outcomes Trial)	19,257	Comparison of two blood pressure treatments
A-HeFT (African-American Heart Failure Trial)	1,050	To determine if a specific medication improves heart failure outcomes in African Americans
CARE-HF (Cardiac Re-synchronization Heart Failure Trial)	813	To determine if cardiac resynchronization improves symptoms and survival in patients with advanced heart failure
CHARM-ADDED (Candesartan in Heart—Failure Assessment of Reduction in Mortality and Morbidity)	2,548	To determine if the addition of an ARB to an ACE inhibitor improves outcome in patients with heart failure
STARRS (Statins for Risk Reduction in Surgery Study)	1,163	To determine if statin use in patients undergoing vascular surgery is of benefit

company that has developed the new treatment or diagnostic test. Large trials also may be supported by other nonindustrial sources such as the National Institutes of Health or other funding agencies. Before it begins, the study must be reviewed by an ethical review committee to fully evaluate both its potential risks to participants as well as its scientific merit.

Large clinical trials are generally required before the Food and Drug Administration (FDA) considers a new form of treatment—either drugs or devices. Moreover, only after the FDA approves such a treatment will it be produced and marketed commercially. In the FDA's Phase I studies, which are small trials designed to evaluate safety in humans (and which are conducted generally only after safety in other animals has been established), a small group of normal subjects is involved. In Phase II studies, which involve actual patients, optimal doses are established and preliminary evidence is gathered of the drug's or device's possible benefit. Phase III studies are the large clinical trials designed to demonstrate clinical efficacy. These are generally key to FDA approval, and they are usually done to compare the new therapy to existing and accepted treatments or, when appropriate, a placebo. Finally, in Phase IV trials, which are generally carried out after FDA approval, further aspects of the new treatment are explored, such as additional indications for use and long-term safety.

WHO PARTICIPATES IN CLINICAL TRIALS?

Clinical trials generally involve large numbers of patients who agree to participate in a study designed either to provide a better understanding of a disease or to provide data concerning the efficacy of a new therapy or diagnostic procedure. Enough patients must be included so that the results are statistically meaningful and can be reasonably applied to the general population. Before the start of a trial, statisticians do what is called a "power" calculation to determine how many patients are needed to establish the treatment's effectiveness. Results are evaluated during the study, and if a treatment is statistically demonstrated to be unequivocally either beneficial or harmful, the trial may be concluded before enrolling the predetermined number of patients.

When patients hear about an experimental drug or procedure, they often want to try it. But not all patients are good candidates to participate in studies because clinical trials are designed to produce reliable answers. Consequently, the criteria for participation are often quite stringent. The investigators running the study must choose those patients who not only have the specific condition, but also are free of confounding medical problems that might influence the results.

Trials are always carried out with patient safety as the highest consideration. In certain trials, a participant may receive a placebo (a "sugar" pill that contains no active ingredients) as opposed to the drug being tested. This may be the only way to know if the new treatment really works. Patients generally do not know whether they are getting the active drug or the placebo, and in most instances, the researchers also do not know which is which. Such a "double-blind study" is intended to remove any bias on the part of the patients and the investigators. In instances in which it is unethical to use a placebo, a new treatment is compared to one that is the current standard of care.

PARTICIPATING IN A CLINICAL TRIAL

Clinical trials may provide your only opportunity to receive the newest drugs or devices before their widespread availability following FDA approval. Although the therapeutic benefit may not be unequivocally established at the time of the trial, there may be good evidence that those who participate are likely to be helped. Consequently, participating in certain clinical trials can give you timely access to cutting-edge therapy that is otherwise unavailable. But not all patients—even those who may clearly be helped by a still-experimental therapy—are good candidates for the study. In such instances, an exception may be made on compassionate grounds to let a very ill person receive an unapproved drug when other alternatives are not helpful.

Of course, in certain trials you may receive the placebo rather than the active form of therapy. The implications of this possibility should be explained fully and clearly by the investigator. It's also important to recognize that a certain percentage of patients benefit from the inactive placebo. This placebo effect, which has puzzled doctors since ancient times, still is not fully understood, but it is generally accepted as further evidence of the influence of the brain on the body. In other words, if a person is convinced that a particular pill or therapy will help, it may often, at least in part, do so, even though there is no direct scientific basis for the benefit.

During a clinical trial, participants may be required to undergo additional diagnostic tests as part of the protocol. These can range from simple blood tests to more extensive diagnostic testing, or even cardiac catheterization. There may be need for follow-up evaluations and periodic telephone calls concerning your overall health status. Blood samples may be stored for future analysis.

In some clinical trials, participants are compensated financially; this also must be defined in advance. You may also receive reimbursement for expenses incurred while participating, such as parking or travel costs. Another benefit for participants is earlier access to the new therapy if the trial is successful: there is often a lag time between completion of the trial and FDA approval, but in most instances, trial participants continue to have access to the new therapy during this period.

INFORMED CONSENT

Everyone who participates in a clinical trial signs an informed consent form, which provides details on all aspects of participation; it also defines precisely any anticipated risks. Read this consent form carefully and ask any questions before signing it. In the past, clinical studies were sometimes conducted in prisons or involved other unwitting individuals. This practice is no longer allowed, and today, informed consent forms are generally quite detailed, often several pages long. The informed consent form, and indeed the entire study, must be approved by a local ethics board prior to the study's launch at that site.

POSSIBLE ETHICAL ISSUES

Participation in a clinical trial or clinical research is purely voluntary. You may choose to participate for a variety of reasons, ranging from gaining access to new therapies to wishing to assist in expanding the knowledge and treatment of a condition that has affected you or a family member. You should never feel coerced or fear that your physician's current treatment will in any way be compromised if you elect not to participate in the trial.

Before enrolling, find out how the trial is being supported. For example, is it being paid for by a pharmaceutical company, a government agency, or a research institution? Try to determine whether there may be any conflict of interest by either those seeking your enrollment or those leading this study.

SUMMING UP

Clinical trials are a key to expanding our knowledge and advancing medical care for the good of all. No matter how convincing a new treatment appears in experiments and in experimental animals, it must be proven to aid significant numbers of patients before it can be accepted as a safe addition to our other therapeutic choices. Our cautions in this chapter are by no means intended to discourage participation in clinical trials; rather, we feel it is important for you to have some understanding of clinical trials, what they are, what's involved, and what you will be asked to do if you do choose to participate. The many checks and balances employed in clinical trials, as well as the rigor with which these trials are undertaken and evaluated, should give everyone involved with heart care—patients, families, and health-care providers—confidence that the latest and best innovations, if found effective and safe, will soon be available for all patients who can benefit from them.

T hroughout this book, we described short case histories that illustrate the type of problems faced by heart patients. Virtually all patients will experience occasional lapses and setbacks, and our sample patients are no different. Stanley, the fifty-five-year-old executive, continues to work long hours but he is more diligent about taking the medications to control his high blood pressure and elevated cholesterol. He also has kept his weight down to around normal. After undergoing knee-replacement surgery, rehab, and physical therapy, he again can work out at his gym without suffering severe knee pain. When he's not on a business trip, he enjoys long walks with his wife.

Alice, the forty-five-year-old school aid, is still a bit overweight, but her diabetes is under control. She has increased her exercise regimen to thirty to forty minutes almost every day. Jennifer, the fifty-year-old long-distance runner, has had no further episodes of chest pain following her angioplasty and stent procedure. The statin drug her doctor prescribed has lowered her blood cholesterol levels to normal. She continues to run, but has given up marathons in favor of shorter five- or ten-kilometer runs. Although these events aren't as thrilling as marathons, they provide an outlet for her competitive drive. She recently bought a mountain bike and looks forward to weekend outings with a biking group.

After two or three lapses, Sam, the fifty-two-year-old school bus driver, has managed to stay off cigarettes. Weaning himself off the nicotine substitutes has been more difficult than he anticipated, and during stressful times, he has resorted to smoking a cigarette or two. But all in all, he's in much better shape than when he first sought medical attention for chest pains. Medication keeps his blood pressure and diabetes under control. His weight has dropped to near normal and he continues to walk his dog for thirty minutes or more twice a day. At his last checkup, his cholesterol was in the normal range, thanks to his increased exercise, weight loss, and a cholesterol-lowering medication.

John, the eighty-five-year-old retiree, continues to do well after coronary by-pass surgery and cardiac rehab. He plays golf two or three times a week and also takes daily walks with his wife of sixty years. He's certainly living proof that you're never to old to undergo cardiac treatment, including surgery and lifestyle changes.

Not all patient stories will have such happy endings, and in the coming years, these patients are likely to endure a progression of their heart conditions. But without a doubt, they all enjoy an improved quality of life and can look forward to more years of relative good health. All have established good working relationships with their physicians, and all agree that their altered lifestyles have given them a renewed sense of empowerment. Without qualification, we can say that what has worked so well for these patients can also work for you.

We expect that different portions of this book will have special relevance for different individuals. As a whole, the book is meant to provide you with a framework on which to build a body of knowledge and a way in which to develop guiding principles that will enhance your long-term health maintenance and care. Much as in the teaching of medical students, defining an approach to the problem is at least as significant as learning its specifics. While the information on heart care presented in this book can be a means to individual empowerment, it is only a first step—not only because heart therapies are evolving so rapidly, but also because your overall mindset is equally important to your continued success. As you cooperate fully with doctors and other medical professionals, look for opportunities to be more active physically, find a diet that is nutritious and fits your lifestyle, and be open to trying new ways to improve your health and outlook as your situation changes. In so doing, you can expect to enjoy a longer and healthier life. Ultimately, it's not what's in the book; it's how what's in the book is used. In that spirit, we hope you will use the insights presented here to improve your health and the health of those you care for.

ACKNOWLEDGMENTS

Many individuals helped in the preparation of this book. Our editor, Jean Thomson Black of Yale University Press, provided invaluable advice and support throughout this creative process. Her detailed review of the initial manuscript greatly improved the final product, as did that of Jenya Weinreb, also of Yale University Press. Our copy editor, Julie Carlson, did a masterful job of putting the final touches on the manuscript.

We acknowledge the talent and diligence of our illustrator, Wendolyn B. Hill. Daron Gardner helped to process the ECG and echocardiography illustrations.

The superb effort of Astrid Swanson in the preparation of this manuscript is gratefully appreciated. Without her skill and dedication this book could not have been written.

Several colleagues provided assistance. Drs. Stephen Possick and David Litvak provided some key reference material. Dr. Lynda E. Rosenfeld provided an ECG example, and Dr. Gaby Weissman provided the echocardiographic images. Dr. William P. Batsford reviewed a portion of the manuscript. Dr. James Perry provided valuable input concerning centers for adults with congenital heart disease.

Finally, without the patience and support of our respective spouses, Myrna and Gerald, this undertaking would not have been possible.

ablation   A technique in which a small amount of heart tissue is destroyed to treat an abnormal heart rhythm.

acute mountain sickness   A disease that develops in some people traveling from a low to high altitude.

aneurysm   An outward bulging, or protrusion, in a blood vessel due to a weakness in the vessel wall; often affects the aorta.

angina pectoris   Pressure or pain due to reduced blood flow to the heart muscle. Pain is typically felt in the middle of the chest, but it may radiate to the back, abdomen, arms, or jaw.

angiogram   An X-ray movie of the coronary arteries, other blood vessels, or other parts of the cardiovascular system.

angiography   Diagnostic procedure in which a dye is injected into the circulation to make blood vessels or parts of the heart visible on X-rays.

angioplasty   Interventional cardiology procedure in which a balloon-tipped catheter is inserted into a narrowed artery and the balloon is then inflated at the site of narrowing to widen the vessel channel.

angiotensin   A natural blood chemical that constricts, or narrows, blood vessels, thus raising blood pressure.

angiotensin-converting enzyme (ACE) inhibitors   Antihypertensive drugs that reduce the action of angiotensin, thereby lowering blood pressure.

ankle/brachial index   A diagnostic study in which the blood pressures in the arm (brachial) and lower leg are measured; it is intended to detect occluded arteries in the legs.

anomalous pulmonary venous drainage   A congenital defect in which one or more of the pulmonary veins drain into the right atrium instead of the left atrium.

antiarrhythmics   A class of drugs used to control abnormal heart rhythms.

anticoagulants   A class of drugs that suppress the body's blood-clotting process.

antihypertensives   A class of drugs that lower high blood pressure.

aorta   The body's largest artery; it arises from the heart's left ventricle and branches to supply blood to the upper body and abdomen.

aorta–left ventricular fistula   An abnormal connection between the first portion of the aorta and the left ventricle.

aortic regurgitation or insufficiency   Failure of the aortic valve to close properly, allowing a backflow of blood into the left ventricle instead of being forced into the aorta.

aortic stenosis   A stiffness or narrowing of the aortic valve, resulting in obstructed blood flow and an increased workload for the heart.

aortic valve   The valve that controls blood flow from the left ventricle, the heart's major pumping chamber, and the aorta, the body's largest artery that arises from the heart.

arrhythmia   Abnormal heartbeat, usually due to an abnormality in the heart's electrical system.

arteries   Blood vessels that carry oxygenated blood from the heart to all parts of the body.

arterioles   The smallest arteries; they distribute oxygenated blood to the capillaries, which in turn nourish the individual cells.

arteriosclerosis   A condition commonly referred to as "hardening of the arteries," in which the artery walls thicken and lose elasticity. Often used synonymously with atherosclerosis.

atherosclerosis   Stiffening or loss of elasticity of arteries due to a buildup of fatty deposits (plaque).

atrial fibrillation   Abnormal heart rhythm in which the heart's upper chambers beat at an excessive or irregular rate.

atrial flutter   A rhythm disorder in which abnormal beats travel in cycles around the atrium, resulting in a very rapid heartbeat.

atrial septal defect   Congenital abnormality resulting in a persistent opening between the left and right atria.

atrial septum   The thin wall dividing the heart's upper chambers (atria).

atrioventricular (AV) node   The small mass of conduction tissue between the heart's upper and lower chambers. The electrical impulses passing through the node control the heart's rhythm.

atrium (plural: atria)   The upper heart chambers. The right atrium receives oxygen-depleted blood from the venous system; the left atrium receives freshly oxygenated blood from the lungs.

automated external defibrillator (AED)   Compact portable device that can administer an electrical shock to the heart; used to treat sudden cardiac arrest.

beta blockers   A class of medications that inhibit the beta-adrenergic nerve receptors; they are used to treat angina, high blood pressure, and cardiac arrhythmias.

blood pressure   The force that blood exerts on the artery walls as it is pumped through the body. It is stated in two numbers, such as 120/80; the first number represents the systolic pressure, the maximum force exerted when the heart pumps out blood, and the second number represents the diastolic pressure, which occurs as the heart momentarily rests between beats.

bradycardia   An abnormally slow heartbeat, typically less than sixty beats per minute in adults.

calcium channel blockers   A class of drugs that inhibit the action of calcium on the artery muscles, thereby lessening the degree of contraction; they are used to treat angina, hypertension, cardiac arrhythmias, and other cardiovascular disorders.

capillaries   The microscopic blood vessels that supply oxygen and nutrients to the cells and pick up carbon dioxide and other waste products to remove from the body.

cardiac arrest   Catastrophic event in which the heart stops beating, resulting in loss of consciousness and death if allowed to persist for more than a few minutes; usually caused by ventricular fibrillation, a condition in which the heart quivers instead of beating normally.

cardiac catheterization   A procedure in which a catheter is inserted into a blood vessel, often an artery in the groin, and threaded through the circulation to the heart. A dye may then be injected to make the heart's blood vessels and other structures visible on X-rays. Various therapeutic interventions may also be carried out during cardiac catheterization.

cardiomyopathy   Any disease affecting the heart muscle, often resulting in heart failure.

cardioversion   Use of an electrical shock to restore normal heart rhythm (*see also* defibrillation).

cholesterol   A fatty substance (lipid) essential for many bodily functions. It is both manufactured in the body and consumed from animal products in the diet, and it travels through the bloodstream attached to a lipid-carrying protein (lipoprotein). There are two major types of lipoproteins: high-density lipoprotein (HDL), referred to as the "good" cholesterol, and low-density lipoprotein (LDL), the "bad" cholesterol. Excessive cholesterol, especially LDL, in the blood can lead to a buildup of fatty plaque in the arteries.

coarctation of the aorta   A congenital defect that is associated with the narrowing of the aorta in the abdomen. This condition results in hypertension.

computed tomographic angiography   A diagnostic study in which a contrast substance is injected into the circulation and its movement is then tracked by a tomographic X-ray device; this technique provides a three-dimensional image of the heart and blood vessels.

computed tomographic calcium scoring   A diagnostic study that allows visualization of calcium deposits in the blood vessels, especially the coronary arteries.

conduits   A portion of the surgical therapy for very complex congenital heart disease involving the transport of blood within the cardiovascular system.

congestive heart failure   A condition in which the heart cannot pump enough blood to meet the body's needs. As fluid accumulates in the lungs and other body tissues, swelling (edema) and difficulty in breathing usually result.

constants   Core set of medical values used in the diagnosis and treatment of cardiovascular and other diseases.

coronary artery disease (CAD)   Disease of the arteries that supply blood to the heart muscle.

coronary atherectomy   A procedure done during angioplasty in which fatty deposits (plaque) are cut away and removed.

coronary bypass surgery   A surgical procedure in which blood vessels from elsewhere in the body are grafted onto the heart to bypass blocked portions of the
coronary arteries.

C-reactive protein (CRP)   A protein in blood serum that indicates inflammation in
the body; high levels may be a cardiovascular risk factor.

cyanosis A bluish or purplish discoloration of the skin, caused by the blood receiving inadequate oxygen.

defibrillation   Administration of an electrical shock to the heart to restore a heartbeat after a cardiac arrest or to stabilize a heart rhythm.

diastolic   The second of the two numbers recorded in a blood pressure reading; it
represents the pressure on the artery walls when the heart's pumping chambers
rest momentarily between beats.

dissecting aneurysm   A condition in which blood is forced through a tear in an
artery's inner wall, causing an outward bulge in the vessel.

diuretics   A class of medications that increase the kidney's excretion of sodium and
fluid; these are used to treat high blood pressure, heart failure, and edema.

double outlet ventricle   A complex congenital defect in which both the aorta and
pulmonary artery arise from one rather than two ventricles.

drug-eluting stents   Stents are devices inserted into blood vessels to prevent renarrowing following angioplasty; drug-eluting stents are impregnated with substances that prevent cell growth from the vessel wall into the stent.

ductus arteriosus   A connection between the aorta and left pulmonary artery that
is present in the fetus but normally closes at birth. When it remains open, it results in a significant congenital defect.

dyspnea   Shortness of breath or difficulty breathing.

Ebstein anomaly   A congenital defect of the tricuspid valve that results in insufficiency of the valve and is frequently associated with cardiac arrhythmias.

echocardiogram/echocardiography   A diagnostic procedure that uses high-frequency
(sonar or ultrasound) waves to produce images of the heart's structures.

edema   Swelling due to fluid retention; most often affects the lower limbs.

Eisenmenger syndrome   A very severe form of congenital heart disease associated
with marked elevation of blood pressure in the pulmonary arteries.

ejection fraction   The percentage of blood in the left ventricle that is pumped into
the circulation with each heartbeat.

electrocardiography   A diagnostic procedure that records the heart's electrical
activity and beats; the tracing it produces is called an electrocardiogram (ECG
or EKG).

electrophysiological testing   In this diagnostic study done in a catheterization laboratory, a catheter is guided to the heart and electrodes are used to make detailed recordings of the heart's electrical system and activity.

embolism (plural: emboli)   A clot or other substance that travels through the
bloodstream and can block an artery. Depending on the site of blockage, this
can cause a heart attack, stroke, or pulmonary (lung) embolism.

endarterectomy   A surgical procedure to remove the inner lining of a blood vessel narrowed by fatty deposits.

endocarditis   Inflammation of the interior lining of the heart (endocardium) and heart valves; often caused by a bacterial infection.

endocardium   The inner lining of the heart.

exercise stress test   An electrocardiogram that is done while a person exercises on a treadmill or stationary bicycle.

fibrin   A protein instrumental in blood clotting.

fibrinogen   A blood component necessary for clotting; it is converted by enzymes into fibrin.

Fontan procedure   A surgical procedure for advanced and complex congenital heart disease that redirects blood from the venous system directly to the pulmonary arteries without passing through the usually deformed or obstructed ventricle.

heart block   A malfunction of the electrical system that blocks signals from the atria to the ventricles.

heart failure   A condition in which the heart cannot pump enough blood to meet the body's needs; as fluid accumulates in the lungs and other body tissues, it results in swelling (edema) and difficulty breathing.

heart murmur   An abnormal sound caused by turbulent blood flow due to a defective heart valve or some types of congenital heart disease.

high-density lipoprotein (HDL)   The so-called good cholesterol because it carries excessive cholesterol away from the artery walls and transports it to the liver where it is metabolized (*see also* cholesterol).

Holter monitor   A portable ECG that provides constant monitoring over a twenty-four-hour period or longer.

homocysteine   An amino acid that is a normal part of protein metabolism; high levels appear to increase the risk of heart disease.

hyperlipidemia   Excessive amounts of fats, or lipids, in the blood.

hypertension   The medical term for high blood pressure.

hypertrophic cardiomyopathy   Abnormal increase in the thickness of the heart's walls.

hypoxia   Insufficient levels of oxygen in the body's tissues.

idiopathic hypertrophic subaortic stenosis (IHSS)   A condition marked by excessive stiffness of the heart muscle because of increased muscle mass and obstruction to the flow of blood from the left ventricle; can result in heart failure.

implantable cardioverter defibrillator (ICD)   A small device, like a pacemaker, that is implanted in the chest in order to automatically detect ventricular fibrillation or ventricular tachycardia; if this happens, it administers an electrical shock to restore a normal heartbeat.

intermittent claudication   Sporadic pains in the leg muscles that come on during exercise and subside during rest; caused by narrowed arteries in the legs.

ischemia   A deficiency of oxygen in a body part due to an obstructed blood vessel; when a coronary artery is involved, it can result in angina and other symptoms.

lipoprotein (a) /Lp(a)   A protein molecule that is a component of LDL cholesterol; it prevents the normal dissolving of blood clots, thereby increasing the risk of a heart attack due to a coronary thrombosis.

low-density lipoprotein (LDL)   The so-called "bad" cholesterol. High LDL levels can result in a buildup of fatty deposits in the artery walls.

Marfan syndrome   A rare inherited disease affecting the connective tissues and resulting in abnormalities of the skeleton, heart, and blood vessels.

metabolic syndrome   A constellation of cardiovascular risk factors, including abdominal obesity, elevated triglycerides and low HDL cholesterol levels, high blood pressure, and insulin resistance.

METs   Metabolic equivalents; a measure of energy consumed by various activities.

mitral atresia   A complex congenital defect associated with abnormal development of the mitral valve.

mitral insufficiency/regurgitation   Failure of the mitral valve to close properly, allowing some blood to flow back into the left atrium rather than moving forward into the left ventricle.

mitral valve   The valve that controls flow of oxygenated blood from the left atrium into the left ventricle.

mitral valve prolapse   A condition in which the mitral valve's flaps (leaflets) are larger than normal; it may result in a type of heart murmur and, in unusual cases, mitral insufficiency.

myocardial infarction (MI)   Medical term for a heart attack.

myocarditis   Inflammation of the heart muscle.

myocardium   The heart muscle.

orthostatic hypotension   An abrupt drop in blood pressure that occurs when a person stands up; can result in fainting.

ostium primum atrial septal defect   A complicated form of atrial septal defect in which the communication between the atria occurs in the lower portion of the atrial chambers.

pacemaker   The center of the heart's electrical activity that controls its rhythm; the term also applies to an implanted device used to control an abnormal heart rhythm.

palpitations   A sensation that the heart is pounding; may be caused by an irregular, strong, or rapid heartbeat.

paroxysmal tachycardia   A sudden increase in the heart rate.

patent foramen ovale   A congenital abnormality resulting in incomplete closure of the atrial septum under certain conditions. This abnormality has been associated with strokes, especially in younger individuals.

percutaneous coronary intervention (PCI)   *See* angioplasty.

percutaneous transluminal coronary angioplasty (PTCA)   An interventional cardiology procedure that involves insertion of a balloon-tipped catheter into the coronary arteries (*see also* angioplasty).

perfusion imaging   Diagnostic study using radionuclide scanning to visualize the pattern of blood flow (perfusion) in the heart.

pericardium   The membrane surrounding the heart.

peripartum cardiomyopathy (PPCM)   A type of heart muscle disease that develops during or immediately after pregnancy.

peripheral vascular disease (PVD)   Disease affecting the outlying arteries, especially those in the limbs.

plaque   Fatty deposits in the inner lining of the arteries (*see also* atherosclerosis).

positron emission tomography (PET) scanning   A diagnostic test using special radioisotopes that emit positrons and produce three-dimensional scans of the heart's blood flow and function.

potassium   A mineral (electrolyte) essential in maintaining the body's chemical balance and proper muscle function.

premature ventricular contractions (PVCs)   Extra or early heartbeats originating in the ventricle.

primary pulmonary hypertension (PPH)   High blood pressure affecting arteries of the lungs.

pulmonary atresia   A condition in which the pulmonary valve and/or pulmonary vasculature does not develop.

pulmonary regurgitation/insufficiency   A defect of the pulmonary valve that allows a backflow of blood into the right ventricle.

pulmonary stenosis   A narrowing or obstruction of the pulmonary valve or artery that impedes blood flow to the lungs.

pulmonary valve   The valve between the right ventricle and pulmonary artery; oxygen-depleted blood passes through it on its way to receiving more oxygen in the lungs.

pulmonary vascular obstructive disease   A condition that develops in certain kinds of congenital heart disease that feature an increase in blood flow to the lungs. When this develops, there is a marked rise in blood pressure within the lungs.

Purkinje fibers   A network of specialized heart muscle cells that carries electrical impulses to the walls of the heart's ventricles.

radioisotope or radionuclide scanning   Test in which a radioactive substance (isotope) is injected into the circulation and tracked by a gamma camera.

regurgitation   Backflow of blood through a valve that does not close properly.

restenosis   Recurrent narrowing or blockage of a blood vessel after treatment such as balloon angioplasty.

revascularization   Growth of new blood vessels.

robotic surgery   Use of a computerized robot to assist in surgery; may be utilized by the on-site operating team or manipulated from a distant location.

saturated fats   Fatty acids that contain the maximum amount of hydrogen. Hard at room temperature and abundant in animal fats and tropical oils (palm, palm kernel, or coconut), they are implicated in the development of hyperlipidemia and coronary artery disease.

septal defect   An imperfection, usually congenital, in which there is an opening in the wall (septum) dividing the heart's left and right sides.

septum   The muscular wall that divides the two halves of the heart. Problems with the septum are often associated with defects of the mitral and tricuspid valves as well as heart block.

sick sinus syndrome   Failure of the sinus node to conduct electrical impulses properly, resulting in a slow heart rate.

single photon emission computed tomography (SPECT)   A diagnostic test that uses radionuclide scanning to produce a three-dimensional image by a camera that rotates around the person being examined.

single ventricle defect   A complex congenital defect in which only one of the two ventricles develops normally.

sinoatrial node   The heart's natural pacemaker; it consists of specialized cells that control the heart's electrical activity.

sinus of Valsalva fistula/aneurysm   A congenital defect resulting from dilation of the sinus of Valsalva, which is above the aortic valve leaflets. If there is a fistula there is a communication to another chamber. If there is only dilation it is called an aneurysm.

sinus venosus atrial septal defect   A kind of atrial septal defect in which the abnormal communication occurs in the upper portion of the atrial septum. This condition is often also associated with abnormal pulmonary venous return.

sleep apnea   Brief periods during sleep in which a person stops breathing normally; this phenomenon has been linked to an increased risk of sudden cardiac death.

sphygmomanometer   The technical name for the device that measures blood pressure.

statins   A class of drugs prescribed to lower high blood cholesterol, especially the "bad" LDL cholesterol.

stem cells   Primitive cells that have the potential of developing into the cells that make up diverse body tissues and organs.

stenosis   Narrowing of a blood vessel, heart valve, or other body passage.

stents   Tiny devices that are inserted into an artery to keep it open.

subvalvular pulmonic stenosis   A narrowing of the blood vessel carrying blood from the pulmonic valve due to either fibrous tissue or increased muscular tissue, causing an obstruction of blood flow to the lungs.

subvalvular or supravalvular aortic stenosis   An obstruction of blood flow from the left ventricle to the aorta either below (subvalvular) or above (supravalvular) the aortic valve.

supraventricular tachycardia   An abnormally fast heartbeat that occurs when the tissue above the ventricles generates impulses at a faster rate than does the heart's usual pacemaker.

surgical ventricular restoration   Surgical procedure to remodel a ventricle damaged by a heart attack or heart failure.

syncope   Medical term for fainting.

systolic   The first of the two numbers in a blood pressure; it corresponds to the pressure exerted on blood vessel walls when the heart contracts.

tachycardia   Rapid heartbeat, typically more than one hundred beats per minute in an adult.

tetralogy of Fallot   A complex congenital defect associated with cyanosis (a blue cast to the skin that indicates inadequate oxygen supply to the blood). The four components of the defect are obstruction to outflow from the right ventricle, thickening from the right ventricular wall, a large ventricular septal defect, and unusual placement of the aorta.

thrombus   A blood clot within the cardiovascular system.

transdermal   A kind of medication delivered through the skin.

transmyocardial laser revascularization   Use of a laser during heart surgery to create small channels within the muscle wall to improve blood flow.

transposition of the great arteries   A congenital condition in which the normal placement of the aorta and pulmonary arteries with respect to the right and left ventricles is reversed. This condition will be incompatible with life unless intervention is performed.

tricuspid atresia   A congenital condition in which the tricuspid valve, which prevents blood from flowing backward into the right atrium from the right ventricle, does not develop.

tricuspid regurgitation or insufficiency   Inability of the tricuspid valve to close properly, allowing a backflow of blood into the right atrium.

tricuspid stenosis   Narrowing or stiffness of the valve between the right atrium and right ventricle.

triglyceride   A fatty substance (lipid) that is found in fatty tissue and also circulates in the blood. High levels may play a role in atherosclerosis.

truncus arteriosus   A complex congenital abnormality in which a single vessel forms the outlet of both ventricles and then gives rise to the aorta and pulmonary arteries. It is always accompanied by a ventricular septal defect.

variables   Individual characteristics that must be considered in designing an appropriate treatment plan.

vascular endothelial growth factor (VEGF)   A chemical substance that can stimulate growth of new blood vessels.

vasoconstriction   The transient constriction or narrowing of a blood vessel.

vasodilator   A substance that causes blood vessels to relax, or dilate.

venous thrombosis   Medical term for blood clots in the veins.

ventricles   The heart's two lower chambers. The right ventricle receives blood from the right atria and pumps it to the lungs; the left ventricle, the heart's major pumping chamber, forces blood into the aorta to circulate through the body.

ventricular assist device   A mechanical device that bolsters the heart's ability to pump blood into circulation.

ventricular fibrillation   A rapid, uncoordinated, or quivering heartbeat that leads to cardiac arrest and death if not corrected.

ventricular septal defect   A congenital abnormality characterized by a persistent opening between the right and left ventricles.

FURTHER READING
AND RESOURCES

Note: Much of the information in this book is based on clinical experience gained over more than thirty years of patient care and scientific research. The sources listed below include basic medical texts and scientific publications.

MEDICAL TEXTS

Sellke F. W., P. J. Dellnido, and S. J. Swanson, eds. *Surgery of the Chest,* 7th ed. Philadelphia: Elsevier Saunders, 2005.

Zipes, Douglas P., Peter Libby, Robert O. Bonow, and Eugene Braunwald, eds. *Braunwald's Heart Disease: A Textbook of Cardiovascular Medicine,* 7th ed. Philadelphia: Elsevier Saunders, 2005.

SCIENTIFIC PUBLICATIONS

Statistics and Risk Factors

American Heart Association: Heart Disease and Stroke Statistics—Update. Dallas: American Heart Association, 2005.

American Society for Bariatric Surgery, "Rationale for the Surgical Treatment of Morbid Obesity." www.asbs.org; updated Nov. 29, 2001.

"Annual Smoking: Attributable Mortality, Years of Potential Life Lost, and Economic Costs—United States, 1995–1999." *MMWR Morbidity and Mortality Weekly Report* 51 (2002): 300.

Centers for Disease Control and Prevention. *Physical Activity and Health: A Report of the Surgeon General.* Washington, D.C.: U.S. Department of Health and Human Services, 1996.

Critchley, J. A., and S. Capewell. "Mortality Risk Reduction Associated with Smoking Cessation in Patients with Coronary Heart Disease: A Systematic Review." *Journal of the American Medical Association* 290 (2002): 86.

Folsom, A. R. E., D. K. Arnett, R. G. Hutchinson, et al. "Physical Activity and Incidence of Coronary Heart Disease in Middle-Aged Women and Men." *Medical Science of Sports Exercise* 29 (1997): 901.

Gaede, P., P. Vedel, N. Larsen, et al. "Multifactorial Intervention and Cardiovascular Disease in Patients with Type 2 Diabetes." *New England Journal of Medicine* 348 (2002): 383.

Garber, A. J. "Attenuating Cardiovascular Risk Factors in Patients with Type 2 Diabetes." *American Family Physician,* Dec. 15, 2000.

Hackam, D. G., and S. S. Anand. "Emerging Risk Factors for Atherosclerotic Vascular Disease: A Critical Review of the Evidence." *Journal of the American Medical Association* 290 (2003): 932.

Libby, P., P. M. Ridker, and A. Maseri. "Inflammation and Atherosclerosis." *Circulation* 105 (2002): 1135.

Malinow, M. R., A. G. Bostom, and R. M. Krauss. "Homocysteine, Diet, and Cardiovascular Disease: A Statement for Healthcare Professionals from the Nutrition Committee." *Circulation* 99 (1999): 178.

Must, A., J. Apadano, E. H. Coakley, et al. "The Disease Burden Associated with Overweight and Obesity." *Journal of the American Medical Association* 282 (1999): 1523.

"Overweight, Obesity, and Health Risk: National Task Force on the Prevention and Treatment of Obesity." *Archives of Internal Medicine* 160 (2000): 898.

Yusuf, S., S. Hawkin, et al. "Effect of Potentially Modifiable Risk Factors Associated with Myocardial Infarction in Fifty-two Countries (the INTERHEART Study): Case Control Study." *Lancet* 364 (2004): 937.

Diet and Alcohol

Goldberg, I. J., L. Mosca, M. R. Piano, et al. "Wine and Your Heart: A Science Advisory for Healthcare Professionals from the Nutrition Committee, Council on Epidemiology and Prevention and Council on Cardiovascular Nursing of the American Heart Association." *Circulation* 103 (2001): 472.

Hu, F. B., and W. C. Willet. "Optimal Diets for Prevention of Coronary Heart Disease." *Journal of the American Medical Association* 288 (2002): 2569.

Ness, A. R., and J. W. Powles. "Fruit and Vegetables and Cardiovascular Disease: A Review." *International Journal of Epidemiology* 26 (1997): 1–13.

Rimm, E. B., P. Williams, K. Fosher, et al. "Moderate Alcohol Intake and Lower Risk of Coronary Heart Disease: Meta-Analysis of Effects on Lipids and Haemostatic Factors." *British Medical Journal* 319 (1999): 1523.

2005 Food Guide Pyramid, MyPyramid.gov, January 2005.

Specific Heart Ailments

Braunwald, E., E. M. Antman, J. W. Beasley, et al. "ACC/AHA 2002 Guidelines Update for the Management of Patients with Unstable Angina and Non-ST-Segment Elevation Myocardial Infarction. Summary Article: A Report of the American College of Cardiology/American Heart Association Task Force on Practice Guidelines." *Journal of the American College of Cardiology* 40 (2002): 1366–1374.

Braunwald, E., and M. R. Bristow. "Congestive Heart Failure: Fifty Years of Progress." *Circulation* 102 (2000): 4–14.

Chobanian, A. V., G. L. Bakris, H. R. Black, et al. "The Seventh Report of the Joint National Committee on Prevention, Detection, Evaluation, and Treatment of High

Blood Pressure: The JNC-7 Report." *Journal of the American Medical Association* 289 (2003): 2560.

Deedwania, P. C. "The Key to Unraveling the Mystery of Mortality in Heart Failure: An Integrated Approach." *Circulation* 107 (2003): 1719.

Hajjar, I., and T. Kotchen. "Trends in Prevalence, Awareness, Treatment and Control of Hypertension in the United States, 1988–2000." *Journal of the American Medical Association* 290 (2003): 199.

Ho, K. K., K. M. Anderson, W. B. Kannel, et al. "Survival after the Onset of Congestive Heart Failure in Framingham Heart Study Subjects." *Circulation* 88 (1993): 107.

Heart Disease in Women, the Elderly, Young Athletes, and Adults with Congenital Heart Disease

Albert, C. M., C. U. Chae, K. M. Rexrode, et al. "Phobic Anxiety and Risk of Coronary Heart Disease and Sudden Cardiac Death among Women." *Circulation* 111 (2005): 480.

Firoozi, S., S. Sharma, and W. J. McKenna. "Risk of Competitive Sport in Young Athletes with Heart Disease." *Heart* 89 (2003): 710–714.

Kannel, W. B. "The Framingham Study: Historical Insight on the Impact of Cardiovascular Risk Factors in Men vs. Women." *Journal of Gender Specific Medicine* 5 (2002): 27.

Lakatta, E., and D. Levy. "Arterial and Cardiac Aging, Parts I, II, and III." *Circulation* 107 (2003): 139.

Manson, J. E., P. Greenland, A. Z. LaCroix, et al. "Walking Compared with Vigorous Exercise for the Prevention of Cardiovascular Events in Women." *New England Journal of Medicine* 347 (1997): 716.

Marron, B. J. "Sudden Death in Athletes." *New England Journal of Medicine* 349 (2003): 1064.

Mikkola, T. S., and T. B. Clarkson. "Estrogen Replacement Therapy, Atherosclerosis, and Vascular Function." *Cardiovascular Research* 53 (2002): 605.

Possick, S. E., and M. Barry. "Evaluation and Management of the Cardiovascular Patient Embarking on Air Travel." *Annals of Internal Medicine* 141 (2004): 148.

Thirty-second Bethesda Conference, "Care of the Adult with Congenital Heart Disease." *Journal of the American College of Cardiology* 37 (2001): 1162.

"Thirty-sixth Bethesda Conference on Eligibility Recommendations for Competitive Athletes in Cardiovascular Abnormalities." *Journal of the American College of Cardiology* 45 (2004): 1322.

Wenger, N. K. "Coronary Heart Disease and Women: Magnitude of the Problem." *Cardiology Review* 10 (2002): 211.

Scientific Advances

Anversa P., M. A. Sussman, and R. Bolli. "Molecular Genetic Advances in Cardiovascular Medicine." *Circulation* 109 (2004): 2832.

Melo L. G., A. S. Pachori, D. Kong, et al. "Molecular and Cell-Based Therapies for Protection, Rescue and Repair of the Ischemic Myocardium." *Circulation* 109 (2004): 2386.

Perin, E. C., Y. J. Geng, and J. T. Willerson, "Adult Stem Cell Therapy in Perspective." *Circulation* 107 (2003): 935.

RESOURCES

Organizations, Addresses, and Web Sites

American Diabetes Association
1701 North Beauregard Street
Alexandria, VA 22311
www.diabetes.org

American Heart Association
320 Greenville Avenue
Dallas, TX 75231
www.americanheart.org

American Society for Bariatric Surgery
7328 West University Avenue, Suite F
Gainesville, FL 32607
www.asbs.org

Centers of Disease Control and Prevention
1800 Clifton Road
Atlanta, GA 30333
www.cdc.gov

National Center for Health Promotion and Disease Prevention
3022 Croasdaile Drive, Suite 200
Durham, NC 277705
www.nchpdp.med.va.gov

National Heart, Lung and Blood Institute
National Institutes of Health
7200 Wisconsin Avenue
Bethesda, MD 20814
www.nhlbi.nih.gov

BOOKS

General

American Heart Association. *American Heart Association Guide to Heart Attack Treatment, Recovery, and Prevention.* New York: Clarkson Potter, 1998.

Groopman, Jerome. *The Anatomy of Hope: How People Prevail in the Face of Illness.* New York: Random House, 2003.

Herbert, Victor, and Genell Subak-Sharpe, eds. *Total Nutrition: The Only Guide You'll Ever Need.* New York: St. Martin's Press, 1995.

Nelson, Miriam, Alice Lichtenstein, and Lawrence Linder. *Strong Women, Strong Hearts.* New York: Putnam, 2005.

Nelson, Miriam, and Sarah Wernick. *Strong Women Stay Young (Revised).* New York: Bantam, 2004.

Roberts, Arthur, Mary O'Brien, and Genell Subak-Sharpe. *Nutraceuticals: The Complete Encyclopedia of Supplements, Herbs, Vitamins, and Healing Foods.* New York: Penguin Putnam, 2001.

U.S. Department of Health and Human Services. *Physical Activity and Health: A Report of the Surgeon General.* Sudbury, Mass.: Jones & Bartlett, 1998.

Diet Books

Agatston, Arthur. *The South Beach Diet: Delicious Doctor-Devised Foolproof Plan for Fast and Healthy Weight Loss.* Emmaus, Pa.: Rodale, 2003.

Atkins, Robert C. *Dr. Atkins' New Diet Revolution (Revised).* New York: M. Evans, 2003.

Barnard, Neal. *Turn Off the Fat Genes: The Revolutionary Guide to Losing Weight.* New York: Three Rivers Press, 2001.

Craig, Jenny. *Jenny Craig's What Have You Got to Lose: A Personalized Weight Management Program.* New York: Villard, 1992.

Rippe, James. *Weight Watchers Weight Loss That Lasts.* New York: John Wiley & Sons, 2001.

Sanders, Lisa. *The Perfect Fit Diet.* Emmaus, Pa.: Rodale, 2004.

Sears, Barry, and Bill Lawren. *The Zone: A Dietary Road Map to Lose Weight Permanently.* New York: ReganBooks, 1995.

abdomen, 19, 101
abdominal fat, 9–10, 61, 171
ABI. *See* ankle/brachial index
ablation, 247
   cardiac arrhythmias and, 143, 145,
      147, 225
   septal, 224
ACE (angiotensin converting enzyme)
   inhibitors, 126, 139, 151, 190, 247
acetazolamide, 211
ACS (acute coronary syndrome), 131
acupuncture, 154
   smoking cessation and, 86, 90
acute coronary syndrome, 131
acute mountain sickness, 211, 212, 247
acute myocardial infarction, 131
adenoids, removal of, 15
adenosine, 110
adolescents
   obesity and, 51
   smoking and, 84
   See also young athletes
adrenal glands, 70, 121, 123
adrenal (stress) hormones, 70, 78, 127
adrenaline, 78, 180
adult congenital heart disease, 199–205
   centers specializing in, 205
AEDs. *See* automated external defibrillators
aerobic exercise, 32, 35, 40, 43, 45, 49
African Americans, 167, 186–88
   antihypertensive drugs and, 190
   diabetes and, 7, 170, 188

diuretics and, 125, 187, 190
heart failure and, 188, 190
heart risk factors for, 5
high blood pressure and, 5, 7, 124,
   125, 187, 188
obesity and, 7, 10, 170, 187–88
salt sensitivity and, 5, 7, 66, 124, 187
treatment considerations for, 190
young athletes' sudden deaths, 195
Agatston, Arthur, 54, 62
age
   cholesterol and, 3, 6, 135
   exercise considerations and, 3, 32,
      34–35, 45, 49
   fibrinogen levels and, 13, 181
   as heart risk factor, 2, 3–4
   heart-valve disease and, 150
   obesity and, 10
   smoking and, 10
   See also elderly people; young athletes
AHA. *See* American Heart Association
airlines, 206, 207
air travel, 206–9
Albert, Christine M., 81
alcoholic beverages, 56
   air travel and, 208
   heart failure and, 141
   high-altitudes and, 211
   moderate wine consumption and,
      65–66, 158
   smoking cessation medications and,
      87
alcoholism, heart failure linked with, 136

alderosterone blockers, 140
allergies, 19, 113–14
aloe vera, 162
alpha-blockers, 127
alternative and complementary thera-
    pies, 154–64
  safety concerns and, 155, 156, 162,
    163, 164
  smoking cessation and, 86, 87, 90
  See also herbal remedies
altitude changes, 206, 210–12
  exercise and, 47, 210–12
altitude sickness, 210–12
ambulatory ECGs. See Holter monitors
American Cancer Society, 90
American College of Cardiology, 21
American Heart Association, 10, 45, 61,
    64, 66, 90, 152, 170, 192
American Medical Association, 21
American Society for Bariatric Surgery,
    58, 59
amiodarone, 145
amoxicillin, 152
amphetamines, 58
AMS. See acute mountain sickness
anaerobic exercise, 43, 45, 47, 48
android obesity, 9, 10
anemia
  eating disorders and, 178
  heart failure and, 136
  pregnancy and, 174
aneurysm, 247
  dissecting, 250
  See also aortic aneurysm; left ventric-
    ular aneurysm
aneurysm resection, 218
anger, stress and, 70
anger management training, 74, 76
angina pectoris. See chest pain
angiogenesis, 229
angiogram, 247
angiography, 29, 97, 131, 138, 151
  computed tomographic, 115–16, 249

  description of, 112–14, 247
  MRI/MRA and, 116–17
angioplasty, 110, 134, 228
  air travel and, 207
  as coronary artery disease treatment,
    34, 131–33
  description of, 34, 112–13, 247
  elderly people and, 183
  as heart failure treatment, 140
  high blood pressure and, 127
  recent advances in, 221, 222–23
  women and, 173
  See also stents
angiotensin, 247
angiotensin converting enzyme (ACE)
  inhibitors, 126, 139, 151, 190, 247
angiotensin-receptor blockers, 126, 139,
  190
ankle/brachial index, 118, 247
ankles, swelling of, 19, 101
anomalous pulmonary venous
  drainage, 247
anorexia nervosa, 87, 177–78
antianginal drugs, 131, 132
antiarrhythmic drugs, 145, 152, 247
antibiotics, 120, 150, 152, 156
anticoagulants, 145, 152, 153, 155, 247
antidepressants, 78, 87
antihypertensives, 8, 123–28, 147, 156,
  190
  classes of, 125–28
  variables in selecting, 130
antioxidants, 66, 159
anxiety/anxiety disorders
  cardiovascular problems and, 69, 77,
    78, 79–81
  chest pain from, 17
  exercise and, 29
  medication for, 73
  See also panic attacks
anxiety management training, 74, 76
aorta, 121, 247
  coarctation of, 249

aorta-left ventricular fistula, 247
aortic aneurysm
  diagnostic tests and procedures, 112, 115, 118
  high blood pressure and, 122
  intravascular therapy for, 223
  Marfan syndrome and, 194
aortic regurgitation or insufficiency, 149, 176, 248
aortic stenosis, 149, 150, 152
  definition of, 248
  elderly people and, 183
  pregnant women and, 176
  young athletes and, 195
aortic valve, 147, 150, 223, 248
aphrodisiacs, herbal, 163
apnea, 14–15, 254
apple-shaped persons, 9–10
ARBs. See angiotensin-receptor blockers
aromatherapy, 74, 154, 158
arrhythmia, 3, 142–47
  ablation for, 143, 145, 147, 225
  air travel and, 207
  congenital heart disease and, 203
  depression and, 77–78
  description of, 142–43, 248
  detection of, 103, 105, 114, 143
  drug treatments for, 145, 152, 247
  eating disorders and, 177
  heart failure and, 136
  heart-valve disease and, 150
  herbal products and, 163
  implanted devices and, 117, 145, 209, 226–27
  interventional treatments for, 145–47
  pregnant women and, 176
  symptoms with, 142, 143
  treatment choices for, 146
  treatment goals for, 147
  types of, 143, 144
  ventricular, 203, 207
  as warning sign, 17–18
  young athletes and, 193, 194, 195

arteries, 121, 248. See also blocked coronary arteries; carotid artery; coronary arteries; coronary artery disease
arteriogenesis, 229
arterioles, 121, 126, 127, 248
arteriosclerosis, 117, 248
arthritis
  congenital heart disease and, 203
  elderly people and, 181
  exercise and, 12, 28, 49
  water exercises and, 29
  See also rheumatoid arthritis
artificial hearts, 219
ASBS. See American Society for Bariatric Surgery
ascites, 19
Asian diet, 63, 65
aspirin
  air travelers and, 208
  bleeding and, 155, 173–74
  blood clot prevention and, 131
  See also baby aspirin
asthma, exercise and, 29, 49
atherosclerosis, 129, 248
  cholesterol levels and, 6
  diagnostic tests/procedures for, 101, 116
  elderly people and, 181
  risk factors for, 6, 7, 14, 50
  saturated fats and, 61
  smoking and, 82, 170
  triglycerides and, 101
  women and, 170, 171
athletes, heart disease and. See young athletes
"athlete's heart," 197
athletic shoes, 35–38, 47
Atkins diet, 62–63, 64
atrial fibrillation, 150, 152, 248
  pregnant women and, 176
  treatment advances for, 225
  treatments for, 145, 147
atrial flutter, 176, 225, 248

atrial septal defect, 200, 223, 248, 252, 253
atrial septum, 248
atrioventrical (AV) node, 142, 248
atrium, 148
automated external defibrillator (AED), 196, 207, 248
autonomic nervous system, 126, 127
avoidance, patient's, 73

baby aspirin
    risks of, 155, 174
    women and, 173–74
bacterial endocarditis, 152
bacterial infection, 13
balloon angioplasty. See angioplasty
bariatric surgery, 58–59
Barnard, Neal, 61
basketball, 195
beans, 61
beer, 56
behavior modification, 73–76
Benecol, 158, 160
benign ventricular hypertrophy, 197
Benson, Herbert, 74
benzodiazepines, 87
berries, 158
beta blockers, 78, 248
    African Americans and, 190
    for arrhythmias, 145
    for coronary artery disease, 131
    for heart failure, 139–40
    for high blood pressure, 126
    young athletes and, 197
beta glucans, 160
binge eating, 177–78
biofeedback training, 74, 75
biologically based therapies, 228–38
biologic heart valves, 153
bittersweet chocolate, 159
biventricular pacing, 226
bleeding, baby aspirin therapy and, 155, 174

blocked coronary arteries
    angioplasty for, 34, 110, 112–13,
        131–33, 173, 221, 222
    diagnostic tests/procedures for, 103,
        110, 112
    See also atherosclerosis
blood clots
    air travelers and, 208–9
    anticoagulants and, 145, 152, 153
    aspirin and, 131
    depression and, 78
    diagnostic tests and procedures,
        112
    drugs dissolving, 173
    fibrinogen and, 13, 82
    functional foods and, 158, 159
    inflammation and, 14
    women's risk factors for, 170
blood disorders
    anemia, 136, 174, 178
    eating disorders and, 178
blood pressure, 248
    low, 178
    normal, 123
    See also high blood pressure
blood pressure measurement, 97, 99,
    122
    by patients, 124, 125
    systolic/diastolic readings from, 122,
        248, 250
    See also high blood pressure
blood sugar, 8, 9, 50, 62, 158
blood tests, 101–3, 135, 138, 183
blood thinners. See anticoagulants
blood vessels
    diagnostic tests/procedures for, 101,
        115, 116, 117–18
    growing of new, 228–32, 253
    high blood pressure and, 122
blue cohosh, 157
BMI (body mass index), 51
    calculation of, 52
    morbid obesity and, 58

overweight/obesity definitions and, 9, 50, 187
body fat. *See* fat (body)
body shape, 9–10, 61, 171
bone loss. *See* osteoporosis
bone marrow, 230, 231, 232, 234
borage oil, 155
brachytherapy, 222
bradyarrhythmias, 143
bradycardia, 177, 248
brain, 122
    mind-body connection and, 81, 216
breast cancer, 4–5, 169
breathing problems. *See* shortness of breath; sleep apnea
Brody, Jane, 55
Brugada syndrome, 194–95, 196, 226
bruises, 155
bulimia, 87, 177–78
buproprion, 87
B vitamins, 14
bypass surgery. *See* coronary bypass surgery

CAD. *See* coronary artery disease
caffeine, 99, 125, 141, 159
calcific degeneration, 150
calcium
    deficiency of, 187
    imbalance in, 177
calcium channel blockers, 19, 248–49
    African Americans and, 190
    for arrhythmias, 145
    for coronary artery disease, 131
    for high blood pressure, 126
calcium deposits, 129, 150
    computed tomographic visualization of, 116
calcium supplements, 156, 158
calisthenics, 43
calorie-counter diets, 64
calories
    in alcoholic beverages, 66

burning of, 41–44, 45
    weight loss and, 59–60, 64
cancer risk, 87, 115, 231
    excess weight and, 50
    fatal heart attack risk for women vs., 4–5, 169
    hormone replacement therapy and, 171
    smoking and, 82, 83
canned foods, 68, 124
canola oil, 61
capillaries, 121, 249
carbohydrates, 62–63
carbon monoxide, 82, 83
cardiac arrest, 129
    definition of, 249
    eating disorders and, 177, 178
    See also sudden cardiac death
cardiac arrhythmia. *See* arrhythmia
cardiac catheterization, 97, 138, 151, 223
    description of, 112–14, 249
cardiac rehabilitation program
    behavior modification and, 74
    exercise and, 31, 35, 46, 141
    group therapy and, 73
    women and, 173
cardiac restructuring, 229
cardiac resynchronization therapy, 140, 226
cardiac ultrasound. *See* resting echocardiography
cardiologists, 21, 78, 203, 204
cardiomyopathy, 249
    heart failure and, 136
    hypertrophic, 136, 193, 195, 196, 224
    peripartum, 136, 175
    right ventricular, 194
    ventricular tachycardia and, 226
    young athletes and, 193, 194, 195, 224
cardiovascular disease. *See* heart disease
cardiovascular physical exams, 99, 101

cardioversion, 249. *See also* defibrillation

"Care of the Adult with Congenital Heart Disease" (Bethesda Conference, 2000), 199–200, 204

carotid artery, 101, 108, 222–23

cashew oil, 61

catheter ablation, 225

catheterization. *See* cardiac catheterization

Centers for Disease Control and Prevention, 9, 51, 77

centrally acting drugs, 127

checkups
  heart disease screening and, 15
  medical histories and, 99
  pre-exercise, 44–45

chest pain (angina pectoris)
  air travel and, 206
  cardiac arrhythmia and, 143
  as coronary artery disease symptom, 131
  description of, 16, 247
  diagnostic tests and, 112
  drug treatments and, 124, 126, 131
  during exercise, 34, 46
  exercise benefits and, 31
  gender differences in, 4
  high CRP level and, 14
  misdiagnosis of, 172–73
  peripartum, 175
  possible causes of, 17
  smoking and, 82
  stress and, 70
  treatment advances for, 224–25
  as warning sign, 16–17
  women and, 4, 172–73

chest trauma, 193–94

chest X-rays, 97, 138, 151

chewing tobacco, 86–87

childhood obesity, 51, 53

Chinese medicine, 154–55

chocolate, 55, 158
  health benefits of, 159

cholesterol
  age and, 3, 6, 135
  body fat and, 61
  coronary artery disease and, 6, 7, 131, 135
  definition of, 249
  depression and, 78
  diagnostic tests and, 101, 135
  diet and, 6, 50, 62–63, 135, 158
  dietary fats and, 61
  drug treatment for, 7, 31, 135, 137, 152, 231, 254
  eating disorders and, 178
  elderly people and, 135, 181
  elevated, 134–36
  exercise and, 31, 45, 135
  functional foods and, 158
  function of, 134
  heart failure and, 141
  as heart risk factor, 2, 3, 5, 6–7
  low-carbohydrate diets and, 62–63
  obesity and, 188
  smoking and, 82, 170
  treatment goals and, 136
  types of, 249, 251
  women and, 171

chordae tendineae, 147

Cialis, 163

cigarettes. *See* smoking

cinnamon, 160

circulatory disorders, 10, 38, 101

clindamycin, 152

clinical trials, 230, 234, 239–43

clopidogrel, 100

clot-dissolving drugs, 173

clothing, exercise, 36, 41, 47

clots. *See* blood clots

cocaine use, 15

cocoa beans, 159

coenzyme Q_{10}, 158, 160

coffee, 56

comfrey, 163

comorbidity, as treatment factor, 28–29

complementary medicine. *See* alternative and complementary therapies

compression stockings, 208, 209

computed tomographic angiography, 115–16, 249

computed tomographic calcium scoring, 116, 249

computed tomography, 127

conduits, 249

congenital heart defects/disease, 167–68, 250
  adults with, 199–205
  arrhythmias and, 203
  cocaine use and, 15
  diagnostic tests/procedures for, 111
  heart failure and, 136, 202
  overview of, 200
  pregnant women and, 176, 203–4
  pulmonary hypertension and, 200, 203
  severity of, 200–202
  specialist care centers for, 205
  treatment options for, 204–5, 251
  unique issues concerning, 203–4
  young athletes and, 193, 196

congestive heart failure, 249
  air travel risks with, 208
  drug treatments for, 126
  heart-valve disease and, 150, 151
  risk factors for, 7, 10
  salt intake and, 66
  smoking and, 10
  stem cell therapy and, 233

constants, 1, 2, 156, 249
  See also risk factors

cool-downs, exercise, 44

coping skills, 76

corn oil, 61

coronary angiography. *See* angiography

coronary arteries
  spontaneous dissection of, 175
  young athlete problems with, 193, 196
  See also blocked coronary arteries; bypass surgery

coronary artery disease (CAD), 70, 129–34
  African Americans and, 187
  air travel and, 207
  antihypertensive medication variables and, 130
  cholesterol levels and, 6, 7, 131, 135
  definition of, 249
  depression and, 77
  diagnostic tests/procedures for, 105–7, 112, 129, 131
  drug treatments for, 131, 132
  eating disorders and, 178
  elderly people and, 181
  erectile dysfunction and, 99
  heart failure and, 136
  heart-valve disease and, 150
  Hispanics and, 189
  lipoprotein (a) and, 13
  Native Americans and, 190
  pre-exercise checkups and, 45
  risk factors for, 5, 13
  smoking and, 82
  South Asians and, 190
  surgical treatments, 131–34, 218
  treatment goals for, 134
  women and, 4, 172
  young athletes and, 195

coronary atherectomy, 222, 249

coronary bypass surgery, 110, 127, 228
  air travel and, 207
  for coronary artery disease, 131, 133
  depression following, 78
  description of, 250
  elderly people and, 183
  for heart attack, 97
  for heart failure, 140
  women and, 173

cortisol, 78

cottonseed oil, 61

"couch potatoes," 12

counseling, 78, 190
  couples, 73

cramps, muscle, 44

C-reactive protein (CRP), 13–14, 250
cross-country skiing, 40, 43
cross training, 38, 40, 182
CRT (cardiac resynchronization
    therapy), 140, 226
CT (computed tomography), 127
Cubans, 189
cultural factors, 30, 167, 186, 190
cyanosis, 176, 200, 203, 250
cycling, 32, 38, 47
cytokines, 231

dairy products, 61
damiana, 163
dancing, aerobic, 40
dark chocolate, 55, 159
deep venous thrombosis, 208–9
defibrillation, definition of, 250
defibrillators
    automated external, 196, 207
    implantable cardioverter, 226–27
    implanted cardiac, 117, 140, 145, 209
dehydration, 177, 178, 211
dementia, 181
denial, 29–30, 73
dental work, heart-valve disease and,
    152
depression, 69, 76–79
    eating disorders and, 178
    exercise and, 32, 78–79
    fatigue and, 19
    heart attacks and, 11, 12, 76–78
    herbal remedies and, 79, 156
    lifestyle changes and, 29
    men and, 77
    sexual dysfunction and, 163
    sources of, 78–79
    stress and, 11
    symptoms of, 79
    women and, 77, 172
diabetes
    African Americans and, 7, 170, 188
    athletic socks and, 38
    coronary artery disease and, 131

diagnostic tests/procedures for, 101
diet and, 9, 61
drug treatments for, 9, 126
elderly people and, 181
erectile dysfunction and, 99, 163
exercise and, 9, 31, 32, 38, 45
heart failure and, 136, 141
as heart risk factor, 8–9
Hispanics and, 189
metabolic syndrome and, 8
Native Americans and, 5, 190
obesity and, 9, 50, 188
triglyceride elevation and, 101
type I and II, 8, 9, 31
women and, 170, 171
diagnostic tests and procedures, 95–119
ankle/brachial index, 118
blood and urine tests, 101–3, 135,
    138, 183
cardiac catheterization, 97, 112–14,
    138, 151
cardiovascular physical exams, 99,
    101
clinical trials, 242
computed tomographic angiography,
    115–16
computed tomographic calcium
    scoring, 116
coronary angiography, 112–14, 131,
    138, 151
C-reactive protein levels, 14
echocardiography, 106, 107–12, 131,
    138, 151, 172
for elderly people, 182
electrophysiological testing, 114, 143
endothelial function testing, 117–18
exercise stress tests, 16, 34, 45, 46,
    105–7, 110, 131, 138, 172
family history and, 5
genetic testing, 119
Holter monitors, 18, 103, 105, 106,
    143
implanted cardiac defibrillator
    follow-up, 117

magnetic resonance imaging and
  angiography, 116–17, 127
medical histories and, 99, 195–98
pacemaker follow-up, 117
positron-emission tomography, 115
tilt-table testing, 114–15
typical progression of, 100–101
vascular ultrasound, 118
young athletes and, 196
See also electrocardiograms
Diamox, 211
diastolic blood pressure, 3, 122, 181,
  250
diastolic heart failure, 136, 181
diazepam, 87
diet and nutrition, 5, 50–68
  age and, 3
  as altitude sickness prevention, 211
  cholesterol levels and, 6, 50, 62–63,
    135, 158
  commonsense approach to, 53–58
  diabetes and, 9, 61
  eating disorders and, 87, 167, 177–78
  elderly people and, 63, 182
  Food Guide Pyramid and, 55, 63, 65
  functional foods and, 155, 158–61
  regional and ethnic diets and,
    63–64
  salt and, 66–68, 187
  ten tips for controlling, 55–57
  wine's benefits and, 65–66, 158
  See also weight loss and control
dietitians, 54
diets. *See* weight loss and control
digestive disorders, 178
digitalis, 140
dilated aortic root, 176
diltiazem, 145
Directory of Medical Specialists, 21
dissecting aneurysm, 250
distal embolic protection devices, 222
distress, 70
diuretics, 124, 125, 139, 151, 187, 190
  definition of, 250

dizziness
  cardiac arrhythmias and, 142, 143
  during exercise, 34, 44, 47
dobutamine, 110
doctors
  changing, 22–23
  choosing, 2, 20–23
  depression treatment and, 78
  exercise program design and, 49
  pre-exercise checkups with, 44–45
  working relationship with, 95–96
  See also specific specialties
dong quai, 157
Doppler ultrasound, 108, 119
double-blind studies, 241
double outlet ventricle, 250
drug-eluting stents, 173, 221, 222, 250
drugs, 154, 228, 229
  age as selection factor, 3–4
  cost of, 184
  elderly people and, 181, 183, 184–85
  interaction concerns and, 79, 131,
    155, 156, 163, 183
  medical histories and, 99, 156
  nonprescription, 99, 183
  pill splitting and, 184
  recent developments in, 217
  remembering to take, 153
  side effects of, 19, 124, 129, 153
  for smoking cessation, 86, 87, 90
  stress reduction and, 73
  traveler concerns with, 209–10
  for weight-loss, 58
  wine consumption and, 66
  See also herbal remedies; *specific
    drugs and drug types*
drug users, infective endocarditis and,
  150
ductus arteriosus, 250
dyspnea. *See* shortness of breath

Eastern medicine, 154–55
eating disorders, 87, 167, 177–78
Eat More, Weigh Less (Ornish), 61, 64

Ebstein anomaly, 250
ECGs. *See* electrocardiograms
echocardiogram/echocardiography,
    106, 107–10, 131, 138, 151
    definition of, 250
    exercise (stress), 109–10, 172
    resting, 107–9
    transesophageal, 111–12
eclampsia, 175
economic factors
    elderly patients and, 184
    lifestyle changes and, 30
    minority populations and, 186, 191
edema, 19, 101, 250
education level, risk factors and, 10
EECP. *See* enhanced external counter-
    pulsation
Eisenmenger syndrome, 250
ejection fraction, 138, 250
EKGs. *See* electrocardiograms
elderly people, 179–85
    category definition of, 179
    cholesterol levels and, 135, 181
    deep venous thrombosis and, 208
    diagnostic tests/procedures and,
        182
    diuretics and, 125
    drug use compliance by, 184–85
    drug use concerns of, 181, 183
    economic considerations for, 184
    exercise and, 34–35, 44, 45, 182
    heart disease and, 20, 167, 179–85
    heart failure and, 136, 181
    heart-valve disease and, 150
    Mediterranean diet and, 63
    salt sensitivity and, 124
    surgical interventions and, 180,
        183–84
electrical cardioversion, 176
electrocardiogram/electrocardiography,
    16, 18, 97, 131, 138, 143, 151
    ambulatory. *See* Holter monitors
    description of, 103, 104, 250
    traveler copies of, 209

women and, 172
    young athletes and, 194, 198
electrocardiographic conditions,
    sudden cardiac death and, 194–95
electrolytes, 41, 66, 177
electrophysiological testing, 114, 143,
    250
electrophysiology, 221, 225
Eligibility Recommendations for Com-
    petitive Athletes with Cardiovascular
    Abnormalities (Bethesda Conference,
    2004), 196
elliptical trainers, 12, 40
embolic stroke, 145
embolism, 145, 250
embryonic stem cells, 232, 233, 234
Enalapril, 151
endarterectomy, 251
endocarditis, 150, 152, 251
endocardium, 251
endomyocardial biopsy, 112
endorphins, 32, 78–79, 159
endothelial function testing, 117–18
endothelial progenitor cells, 230, 231,
    234
endovascular treatment, 223–24
enhanced external counterpulsation,
    224–25
enlarged heart, 150, 151
EPCs (endothelial progenitor cells),
    230, 231, 234
ephedra, 156, 157
epilepsy, 87
EPS. *See* electrophysiological testing
equilibrium radionuclide angiocardiog-
    raphy (ERNA) scanning, 138
erectile dysfunction, 83, 99
erythromycin, 152
essential fatty acids, 160
essential hypertension, 123
estrogen, 4, 170, 171
ethical issues
    clinical trials and, 243
    embryonic stem cells and, 233

ethnic background, 5, 10, 167, 190. *See also specific ethnic groups*
ethnic diets, 63, 65
eustress, 70
exercise, 31–49
    aerobic vs. anaerobic, 32, 35, 40, 43, 45, 47, 49
    age considerations for, 3, 32, 34–35, 45, 49
    benefits of, 12, 31, 43–44, 49
    checkups prior to, 44–45
    cholesterol levels and, 31, 45, 135
    clothing for, 36, 41, 47
    coexisting disorders and, 28–29
    commonsense approach to, 47–48
    cool-downs and, 44
    cross training and, 38, 40, 182
    depression and effects of, 32, 78–79
    diabetes and, 9, 31, 32, 45
    diet and, 51, 63, 68
    after eating, 48
    elderly people and, 34–35, 44, 45, 182
    flexibility training and, 40
    fundamentals of, 41–44
    in groups, 46
    heart failure and, 31, 141
    at high altitudes, 47, 210–12
    high blood pressure and, 31, 45, 123
    model program for, 46, 48
    obesity and, 10, 32, 44
    personalized program design and, 44–46, 49
    program guidelines for, 32–41
    safety concerns and, 41, 47
    strength training and, 36, 40, 45
    stress reduction and, 32, 73
    stretching and, 36, 40, 44, 48
    timing of workouts and, 48
    travelers and, 36, 41, 47, 210–12
    warm-ups and, 40, 44
    water consumption during, 40–41
    weight loss and, 45, 60
    women and, 49, 170
    See also young athletes

exercise echocardiography, 109–10, 172
exercise electrocardiography. *See* exercise stress tests
exercise equipment, 35–36
exercise physiologists, 35, 39, 46, 47, 182
exercise stress tests, 16, 110, 131, 138
    description of, 105–7, 251
    nuclear, 110–11
    pre-exercise checkups and, 45, 46
    target heart rate determination from, 34
    women and, 172
experimental treatments. *See* clinical trials
extracts, 162
eyes
    examination of, 101
    vision loss, 122

FAA. *See* Federal Aviation Administration
fainting (syncope)
    as arrhythmia symptom, 142, 143
    diagnostic tests/procedures for, 114–15
    as warning sign, 18–19, 20
family dynamics, stress and, 72–73
family history
    as heart risk factor, 5
    medical histories and, 99, 195–96
    of smoking, 10
    of young athletes, 195–96
    See also genetics
family physicians, 21, 78
fat (body), 41, 51, 59, 60
    distribution of, 9–10, 61, 171
fat (dietary), 60–61, 64
    saturated, 61, 253
fatigue
    during exercise, 47
    heart failure and, 137
    as warning sign, 19–20
fatty acids. *See* saturated fats
fatty deposits. *See* plaque

FDA. *See* Food and Drug Administration
fear, 27, 73, 215
  panic attacks and, 29, 79–80
  phobic anxiety and, 80, 81
Federal Aviation Administration (FAA), 206, 207
feet
  athletic shoes and, 36–38, 47
  injuries/problems with, 39
Fen-phen (Phentermine and Fenfluramine), 58
fermentation, 162
fertility problems, 83, 178
fetal myocytes, 234
FGF (fibroblast growth factor), 230
fiber, 63, 68
fibrillation. *See* atrial fibrillation; ventricular fibrillation
fibrin, 251
fibrinogen, 13, 82, 181, 251
fibroblast growth factor, 230
field sports, 38
fight-or-flight response, 70, 75
Final Smoke, 87
fingertips, disfigured, 101
fish, 63
fish oil supplements, 155
flavonoids, 158, 159, 160, 162
flavonols, 159
flax, 160
flexibility training, 40
fluoxetine, 78
folic acid, 14, 158
folk medicine, 154
Fontan procedure, 251
Food and Drug Administration, 154, 158, 240–41, 242
food diaries, 54, 57, 60
Food Guide Pyramid, 55, 63, 65
food labels, 56, 66, 68, 124
foods
  salt content in, 67
  See also diet and nutrition

football, 38, 195
foxglove, 157
Framingham Heart Study, 1–2, 5
free weights, 36, 48
freeze-dried extracts, 162
"French factor," 65
fruit juices, 41, 56
fruits, 61, 63
functional foods, 155, 158–61

garlic, 160
gender
  chest-pain sensation and, 4
  depression and, 77
  heart disease prevention/treatment and, 167
  heart disease risk and, 4–5
  smoking and, 11
  young athlete sudden death and, 195
  See also men; women
gene therapy, 228, 236–38
genetic counseling, 204
genetics
  as heart risk factor, 3, 5
  minority groups and, 186, 187, 190
  weight and, 50
  See also family history
genetic testing, 119
geographic factors, lifestyle changes and, 30
gestational hypertension, 175
gingivitis, 87
ginkgo biloba, 155, 156, 161, 212
ginseng, 155, 163
glucomannan, 161
gout, 203
grape juice, 66
green tea, 158
Groopman, Jerome, 215
group exercise, 46
group therapy, 73
growth factors, 229–31, 233
guggul, 161
guided imagery, 76

gum disease, 87
gyms, 36, 41, 47
gynecologists, 21

Habitrol, 86
HACE. *See* high altitude cerebral edema
HAPE. *See* high altitude pulmonary edema
hardening of the arteries. *See* atherosclerosis
Hawaiian natives, 5
hawthorne, 156, 161
HCM. *See* hypertrophic cardiomyopathy
HDL cholesterol (high-density lipoprotein), 135–36
  cholesterol measurement and, 6–7, 135
  diagnostic tests for, 101
  dietary fats and, 61
  exercise and, 31, 45
  as "good" cholesterol, 249, 251
  metabolic syndrome and, 8
  ratio to LDL of, 6–7, 135
  smoking and, 82
  wine drinking, 65–66
  women and, 171
headaches, exercise-related, 47
health care access, 5, 186, 191
health clubs, 36, 41, 47
health maintenance organizations, 21
heart, 122
  age effects on, 180
  anatomy of, 98
  "athlete's," 197
  diagnostic tests/procedures for, 101, 108, 112, 116
heart attack (myocardial infarction), 252
  African Americans and, 187
  air travel and, 206
  anxiety and, 79–80
  cholesterol levels and, 6
  cocaine use and, 15
  coronary artery disease and, 129, 134

depression and, 11, 12, 76–78
diagnostic tests/procedures for, 103
elderly people and, 181
estrogen replacement and, 171
exercise and, 31, 46
exercise fears and, 29
fibrinogen levels and, 13, 82
functional foods and, 158
heart failure and, 136
heart-valve disease and, 150–51
high blood pressure and, 122
high CRP level and, 14
Native Americans and, 190
obesity and, 188
pre-exercise checkups and, 45
psychological factors and, 11, 12, 69
risk factors for, 2–8, 10–15
"silent," 19, 173
smoking and, 10, 82
stem cell therapy and, 236
stress and, 11, 70
surgical ventricular restoration and, 218–19
women and, 4, 80, 170, 171, 173, 175
heart beat. *See* heart rate
heart disease
  anxiety and, 79–81
  congenital. *See* congenital heart defects/disease
  death from, 3, 4, 80, 169, 187, 192–93
  depression and, 77
  in elderly people, 20, 167, 179–85
  exercise and, 31–32, 49
  gender and, 4–5
  individual variation in, 1
  in minority populations, 5, 167, 186–91
  pre-exercise checkups and, 44–45
  preventive treatments and, 120–21
  psychological factors in, 69
  risk factors for, 1–15, 45, 50, 70, 77
  signs and symptoms of, 15–20
  travelers with, 22, 36, 41, 47, 168, 206–12

heart disease (continued)
  wine drinking and, 65–66, 158
  women and, 4–5, 19–20, 77, 167,
    169–78
  young athletes and, 167, 192–98, 224
heart failure, 136–42
  African Americans and, 188, 190
  air travel and, 207
  cardiac resynchronization therapy
    and, 140, 226
  classification of, 139
  congenital heart disease and, 136, 202
  definition of, 136
  device advances for, 219–20
  diagnostic tests/procedures for, 101,
    138
  drug treatment classes for, 141
  drug treatments for, 126, 138–41
  elderly people and, 136, 181
  exercise and, 31, 141
  heart-valve disease and, 136, 150
  high blood pressure and, 122, 136, 141
  new blood vessel growth and, 229
  risk factors for, 7, 136
  salt intake and, 66, 124, 141
  stem cell therapy and, 233–34
  surgical treatments for, 140–41
  treatment goals for, 142
  warning signs/symptoms of, 19
  women and, 181
  See also congestive heart failure
heart-lung machines, 133, 218, 220
heart murmur, 151, 152, 196, 251
heart rate
  arrhythmia symptoms and, 142, 143
  determination of, 33, 34
  diagnostic tests/procedures and, 105,
    107
  exercise and, 33–34, 40, 44
  pulse measurement and, 99
  rapid (tachycardia), 225, 226, 255
  resting, 32, 142
  slow (bradycardia), 146
  "talking pace" and, 44

heart-rate monitors, 33
heart transplants, 140–41, 183–84, 219
heart-valve disease, 111, 147–53
  causes of, 150–51
  common types of, 148–49
  diagnostic tests/procedures for, 151
  drug treatments for, 151–52
  heart failure and, 136, 150
  preventive antibiotic therapy and, 152
  surgical treatments for, 152–53, 220
  treatment advances for, 223–24
  treatment goals for, 153
  valve repair/replacement and, 140,
    153, 224
  valvular insufficiency and, 150
heparin, 145, 209
herbal remedies, 154–58, 160–63
  altitude sickness prevention and, 212
  as aphrodisiacs, 163
  common forms of, 162–63
  dangers of, 157, 163
  depression and, 79, 156
  interaction cautions for, 79, 155, 156,
    163, 183
  medical histories and, 99, 156
  smoking cessation and, 86, 87, 90
high-altitude cerebral edema, 211
high-altitude pulmonary edema, 211
high-altitude travel concerns, 47, 206,
  210–12
high blood pressure (hypertension),
  121–29
  African Americans and, 5, 7, 124,
    125, 187, 188
  age and, 3
  anxiety and, 78
  bulimia and, 178
  cocoa flavonoids' reduction of, 159
  coronary artery disease and, 131
  definition of, 121
  depression and, 77, 78
  diagnostic tests/procedures for, 99,
    101, 122–23
  diet and, 50

drug treatments for, 8, 31, 123–28, 130, 247
elderly people and, 181
exercise and, 31, 45, 123
heart failure and, 122, 136, 141
as heart risk factor, 2, 3, 7–8
heart-valve disease and, 152
Hispanics and, 188, 189
incidence of, 121
interventional treatments of, 127, 129
metabolic syndrome and, 8
Mexican Americans and, 5, 189
Native Americans and, 190
during pregnancy, 170, 174–75
salt and, 61, 66, 123–24, 187
sexual dysfunction and, 163
stress and, 11, 123
treatment goals, 129
weight and, 50, 123
women and, 7–8, 170, 171, 174–75
young athletes and, 196
high-density lipoprotein. See HDL cholesterol
high-dose vitamins, 155, 158
high-fiber supplements, 156
high-protein, low-carb diets, 64
hiking, 38
Hispanics, 5, 10, 167, 188–89
His-Purkinje system, 142
Hollenberg, Norman K., 159
Holter monitors, 18, 103, 105, 106, 143
home blood pressure machines, 124, 125
homeopathy, 155
homocysteine, 14, 158
Hope, Bob, 179
hormone replacement therapy, 4, 170–71, 208
hormones
   blood pressure levels and, 121
   eating disorder effects on, 178
   in herbal products, 163
   stress and, 11, 70, 78
   See also adrenal (stress) hormones; estrogen; insulin

horny goat weed, 163
hotel exercise facilities, 36, 41, 47
HRT (hormone replacement therapy), 4, 170–71, 208
hs-CRP testing, 14
Hyman, Flo, 195
hyperemic response, 117, 118
hypertension. See high blood pressure; pulmonary hypertension
hyperthyroidism, 136
hypertrophic cardiomyopathy, 136, 193, 195, 196, 224
hypertrophy, 103
   benign ventricular, 197
   left ventricular, 7, 181, 188
hypnosis, smoking cessation and, 86, 90

ICDs. See implantable cardioverter-defibrillators; implanted cardiac defibrillators
idiopathic hypertrophic subaortic stenosis (IHSS), 251. See also hypertrophic cardiomyopathy
illness, exercise and, 39, 47
immune system, 70
implantable cardioverter-defibrillators, 226–27, 251
implanted cardiac defibrillators, 117, 140, 145, 209
impotence. See erectile dysfunction
income, as heart risk factor, 5
independence, 73
individualized treatment program, 1–23
   diet and, 50–68
   doctor choice and, 20–23
   exercise and, 31–49
   risk factors and, 3–15
   variables and, 255
   warning signs/symptoms and, 15–20
individual variables, 1, 2, 21, 156
infection, 13, 136, 194
infective endocarditis, 150
inflammation, chronic, 13–14

informed consent, 242–43
infusion therapy, 138
injuries, exercise-related, 39, 43
insulin, 11, 32, 62, 78
insulin resistance, 8–9
intermittent claudication, 251
internists, 21
intravascular ultrasound, 113
iodine, 113
iron supplements, 158
ischemia, 82, 106, 110, 117, 129
    definition of, 251
    myocardial, 70
    silent, 105, 131
isometric exercise, 197. *See also* anaero-
    bic exercise
isoproterenol, 114
isosorbide mononitrate, 163
IVUS (intravascular ultrasound), 113

Jenny Craig, 60
jogging, 32, 36, 40, 41, 43
    shoes for, 37, 38
Johns Hopkins Precursors Study, 77

kidney failure, 7, 122
kidneys, 121, 122, 123
    angioplasty on artery of, 222
    constricted renal arteries and, 127
    diabetes-related damage of, 126
    disorders of, 19, 181

language barriers, minority populations
    and, 190
L-arginine, 161
LDL cholesterol (low-density lipo-
    protein), 13, 135–36
    as "bad" cholesterol, 249, 252
    diagnostic tests for, 101
    dietary fats and, 61
    eating disorders and, 178
    exercise and, 31
    family history and, 5
    high cholesterol diagnosis and, 135

lipoprotein (a) and, 13, 101, 252
    ratio to HDL of, 6–7, 135
    smoking and, 82, 170
    women and, 171
leaflets, 147, 150, 153
lecithin, 161
left ventricular aneurysm, 218
left ventricular hypertrophy, 7, 181, 188
legs
    angioplasty on arteries of, 222
    pain in, 31
    swelling of, 19
    varicose veins in, 19, 38, 208
    See also feet
Levitra, 163
licorice root, 90, 157
lifestyle changes, 95
    complicating factors in, 27–30
    heart failure and, 141
    high blood pressure and, 123–24
    metabolic syndrome and, 8
lifestyle factors
    age and, 3
    elderly people and, 182
    heart failure and, 136
    minority populations and, 190
    sedentary existence and, 12
light-headedness
    as arrhythmia symptom, 142, 143
    during exercise, 46, 47
Lincoln, Abraham, 194
lipid profiles, 101
lipids, 6, 7
lipoprotein (a), 13, 101, 252
lipoproteins, 6, 135. *See also* HDL
    cholesterol; LDL cholesterol
liver disease, 19, 66, 181
lobelia, 157
Long QT syndrome, 194–95, 196, 226
low blood pressure, 178
low-carbohydrate diets, 62–63, 64
low-density lipoprotein. *See* LDL
    cholesterol
low-dose aspirin. *See* baby aspirin

low-fat diets, 60–61, 64
Lp(a). *See* lipoprotein (a)
lung cancer, 82, 83
lungs
    diagnostic tests/procedures for, 101
    fluid retention in, 19
    heart failure and, 136
    See also pulmonary *headings*
LVH. *See* left ventricular hypertrophy

magnetic resonance imaging, angiography and, 116–17, 127
malignant hypertension, 120
MAO inhibitors, 87
Marfan syndrome, 176, 194, 196, 197
massage, 74, 158
meat, 61, 63
mechanical heart valves, 153
Medicaid, 184
MedicAlert bracelets, 41
medical history, 99, 156, 195–98
medical records
    transferring of, 23
    traveling with, 209–10
Medicare, 184
medications. *See* drugs
meditation, 74, 76, 154, 158
Mediterranean diet, 63
memory
    flavonols' improvement of, 159
    problems with, 181, 185
men
    alpha-blockers and, 127
    chest-pain sensation in, 4
    depression and, 77
    erectile dysfunction and, 83, 99
    heart risk factors for, 4
    low-dose aspirin and, 174
    obesity and, 10
    smoking and, 83
    sudden cardiac death and, 4
    young athlete sudden death and, 195
menopause, 4, 10, 83, 171
menstrual cycle, 172, 178

metabolic equivalents, 46
metabolic syndrome, 8, 61, 188, 189, 252
metabolism
    elderly people and, 181, 183
    heart-valve disease and, 150
    individual variation in, 53
    smoking cessation and, 83
    weight loss and, 59, 60, 61, 68
METs (metabolic equivalents), 46, 252
Mexican Americans, 5, 189
MI (myocardial infarction). *See* heart attack
mind-body connection, 81, 216
mineral supplements, 156, 158
minority populations, 5, 7, 167, 186–91
mitral atresia, 252
mitral insufficiency/regurgitation, 148, 150, 151, 176, 252
mitral stenosis, 148, 152–53, 176
mitral valve
    endovascular treatment of, 223
    function of, 98, 147, 252
    heart attack and, 151
    insufficiency of, 150
    surgical repair of, 152–53, 220
mitral valve prolapse, 148, 151, 176, 252
monoamine oxidase (MAO) inhibitors, 87
monounsaturated fats, 61, 63
morbid obesity, 58
mountain sickness. *See* altitude sickness
mouth cancer, 87
MRI/MRA (magnetic resonance imaging), angiography and, 116–17, 127
muscle cramps, 44
MVP (mitral valve prolapse), 148, 151, 176
myocardial infarction (MI). *See* heart attack
myocardial ischemia, 70
myocarditis, 136, 194, 196, 252
myocardium, 152
myxomatous degeneration, 151

National Health and Nutrition Exami-
nation Survey, 77
National Institutes of Health, 4, 240
Native Americans, 5, 167, 189–90
natural remedies. See herbal remedies
nausea, during exercise, 46
Navaho, 190
Nelson, Miriam E., 49
neovascularization, 229
nerve damage, 178
neurocardiogenic syncope, 18, 114–15
New York Heart Association Functional
Classification, 139
NHANES I. See National Health and
Nutrition Examination Survey
Nicocure, 87
Nicoderm CQ, 86
Nicorette, 86
nicotine, 10, 82–90, 125, 170, 211
nicotine gum, 85, 86, 125
nicotine patches, 85, 86
nicotinic acid, 13
nitrates, 131, 139, 190
nitroglycerine, 16, 163, 209
nonprescription drugs, 99, 183
nuclear stress test, 110–11, 131
Nurses' Health Study, 4, 50–51, 80, 171
nutraceuticals, 156, 158, 160–61
nutrition. See diet and nutrition
nutritional supplements, 58, 79, 99, 155.
See also vitamins
nuts, 61

oat bran, 158, 161
obesity
African Americans and, 7, 10, 170,
187–88
BMI (body mass index) definition of,
9, 50, 58, 187
children and, 51, 53
diabetes and, 9, 50, 188
diagnostic tests/procedures and, 111,
112, 115
diet and, 50–51

exercise and, 10, 32, 44
heart failure and, 136
as heart risk factor, 9–10, 50
Hispanics and, 10, 189
metabolic syndrome and, 8, 188
as mortality factor, 50–51
Native Americans and, 190
surgical treatments for, 58–59
women and, 170, 188
See also weight loss and control
obstetricians, 21, 204
Offices for the Aging, 182
olive oil, 61, 63
online physician referral sites, 21
open-heart surgery, 133, 218, 220
optimism, 81
oral contraceptives, 170
Ornish, Dean, 61
orthopedic problems, 12, 28, 47, 181
orthopedists, 39
orthostatic hypotension, 127, 252
orthotics, 37, 38, 39
osteoporosis, 32, 49, 83, 171, 178
ostium primum atrial septal defect, 252
over-the-counter drugs. See nonprescription drugs
overweight, 83, 85
BMI (body mass index) definition of,
9, 50–51
See also obesity; weight loss and
control
oxygen, 41, 121, 129
aerobic exercise and, 32, 43
air traveler concerns about, 207
cyanosis and, 176, 200, 203
metabolic equivalents and, 46
smoking and levels of, 82, 83

pacemaker, 117, 145, 209, 226, 252
pain
exercise and, 39
leg, 31
See also chest pain
pallor, during exercise, 46

palpitations, 17–18, 46, 142, 252

panic attacks, 29, 79–80

paroxetine, 78

paroxysmal tachycardia, 252

pasta, 61, 63

patent foramen ovale, 223, 252

Paxil, 78

PCIs. *See* percutaneous coronary interventions

peanut oil, 61

pear-shaped persons, 10

pediatric cardiologists, 203

peer group support, 190

peer pressure, smoking and, 10–11

penicillin, 152

pennyroyal, 157

percutaneous coronary interventions, 132–33, 221. *See also* angioplasty; stents

percutaneous mitral balloon valvotomy, 223

percutaneous transluminal coronary angioplasty, 252

Perfect Fit Diet, The (Sanders), 53

perfusion imaging, 252

pericardium, 108, 253

peripartum angina, 175

peripartum cardiomyopathy, 136, 175, 253

peripheral vascular disease, 7, 118, 253

personality, 53, 69

pesticides, 162

PET (positron-emission tomography), 115, 253

pets, 73

PFO (patent foramen ovale), 223

pharmaceutical industry, 154, 184

Pheidippides, 192

phlebotomy, 203

phobic anxiety, 80, 81

physical therapists, 47, 49, 182

physicians. *See* doctors

phytochemicals, 66

pill counter/trackers, 185

pill splitting, 184

pituitary glands, 70

placebo effect, 242

placebos, 79, 241, 242

plaque
    angioplasty and, 34
    cholesterol and, 6, 170
    coronary artery disease and, 129
    coronary atherectomy and, 222
    definition of, 253
    inflammation and, 13–14

Plavix, 100

plethysmograph, 117

podiatrists, 39, 47

pokeweed, 157

polyunsaturated fats, 61, 63

Pondimin, 58

population studies, 1–2, 5

portion control, 60, 61, 68

positron-emission tomography (PET) scanning, 115, 253

potassium, 177, 187, 253

potassium channels, 145

PPCM (peripartum cardiomyopathy), 136, 175, 253

PPH (primary pulmonary hypertension), 176, 253

preeclampsia, 175

pregnancy
    cardiovascular system and, 167, 174
    cocaine use during, 15
    congenital heart disease and, 176, 203–4
    heart failure and, 136
    heart problems and, 174–76
    high blood pressure during, 170, 174–75

premature ventricular/atrial beats, 176, 253

primary care physicians, 21, 78

primary pulmonary hypertension, 176, 253

processed foods, 66, 68

pronation, 37, 38

propranolol, 145

protective factors, cardiovascular, 81
protein, 62–63, 64, 68
Prozac, 78, 87
psychiatrists, 78
psychological counseling, 73, 78
psychological factors, 69–81
     heart attack and, 11, 12, 69
     heart health and, 81
     lifestyle changes and, 29
     women and, 171–72
     See also depression; stress
psychologists, 78
psychotherapy, 73
psyllium seed, 161
PTCA (percutaneous transluminal
   coronary angioplasty), 252
Puerto Ricans, 189
puffiness, 19
pulmonary atresia, 253
pulmonary hypertension, 176, 200, 203
pulmonary problems, 29, 82, 247
pulmonary regurgitation/insufficiency,
   149, 253
pulmonary stenosis, 149, 253
pulmonary valve, 147, 152, 223, 253
pulmonary vascular obstructive disease,
   253
pulse measurement, 99, 101, 196
purging, 177–78
Purkinje fibers, 253
PVD (peripheral vascular disease), 7,
   118, 253

racial background, 5, 167, 195. *See also
   specific groups*
racing heartbeat, during exercise, 46
racquetball, 43
radiofrequency catheter ablation, 145, 147
radioisotope/radionuclide scanning,
   172, 253
rebound hypertension, 124
red meat, 61
red rice yeast, 161
Redux, 58

red wine, 65–66, 158
refined starches, 62
reflective clothing, 36, 41
regenerative medicine, 232
regional diets, 63, 65
regional referral centers, 204–5
regurgitation, valvular, 253
     aortic, 149, 176, 248
     mitral, 148, 150, 151, 176, 252
     pulmonary, 149, 253
     tricuspid, 149
rehabilitation. *See* cardiac rehabilitation
   program
relaxation response, 73–74, 75
relaxation techniques, 73–75, 76, 158
resistance exercise. *See* anaerobic
   exercise
resistance exercise machines, 43, 48
restenosis, 132–33, 221, 222, 253
resting echocardiography, 107–9
resting heart rate, 32, 142
resynchronization, heartbeat, 140, 226
revascularization, 253
rheumatic fever, 120, 150, 174
rheumatic heart disease, 120
rheumatoid arthritis, 13
rice, 63
right ventricular cardiomyopathy, 194
risk factors
     heart disease, 1–15, 45, 50, 70, 77
     pre-exercise checkups and, 45
     stroke, 3–8, 10, 14
     target heart rate and, 33, 34
     for women, 4–5, 7–8, 169, 170
robotic surgery, 220, 253
role-playing, 76
Roosevelt, Franklin D., 120
rowing, 43
running, 40, 43, 47, 197
running shoes, 38, 47

safety issues
     alternative/complementary therapies
        and, 155, 156, 162, 163, 164

drug interactions and, 79, 131, 155, 156, 163, 183
exercise and, 41, 47
safflower oil, 61
St. John's wort, 79, 87, 156
salt, 66–68
  content in common foods, 67
  high blood pressure and, 61, 66, 123–24, 187
  tips for cutting back, 68
salt sensitivity
  African Americans and, 5, 7, 66, 124, 187
  elderly people and, 124
Sanders, Lisa, 53, 60
saturated fats, 61
  definition of, 253
secondhand smoke, 10
sedatives, 87
sedentary lifestyle
  exercise and, 36, 39, 43, 45
  as heart risk factor, 12
  women and, 170
seizure disorders, 87
selective serotonin reuptake inhibitors, 78, 87
self-diagnosis/self-treatment, 155, 156
self-esteem, 51, 73
self-hypnosis, smoking cessation and, 86
self-image, exercise and, 32
Selye, Hans, 70
senior centers, 182
septal ablation, 224
septal defect
  atrial, 200, 223, 248, 252, 253
  ventricular, 200
septum, 254
sexual dysfunction. See erectile dysfunction
shoes, athletic, 35–38, 47
shortness of breath (dyspnea), 250
  cardiac arrhythmia and, 143
  coronary artery disease and, 131

during exercise, 34, 46, 47
  heart failure and, 137
  as warning sign, 17
sick sinus syndrome, 254
side effects, drug, 19, 124, 129, 153
sildenafil, 163
silent heart attack, 19, 173
silent ischemia, 105, 131
single photon emission computed tomography, 106, 110–11, 254
single ventricle defect, 254
sinoatrial node, 254
sinus node, 142
sinus of Valsalva fistula/aneurysm, 254
sinus venosus atrial septal defect, 254
ski machines, 40
sleep apnea, 14–15, 254
sleep disorders, 19
sleeping pills, 211
smokeless tobacco, 86–87
SmokEnders, 90
smoking, 50, 82–92
  blood pressure measurement and, 99
  fibrinogen levels and, 13, 82
  heart failure and, 136, 141
  as heart risk factor, 10–11
  nicotine and, 10, 82–90, 125, 170, 211
  quitting of, 10, 11, 83–92
  self-assessment quiz, 88–89
  weight gain and, 11, 83
  by women, 11, 83, 170
smoking cessation program, 90
snacking, 56, 68
snuff, 86–87
soccer, 38, 195
socioeconomic status, 10, 186, 191
soda, 41, 56
sodium. See salt
soft drinks, sugar-free, 56
sotalol, 145
South Asians, 5, 190
South Beach Diet (Agatston), 54, 62, 64
soybeans, 61, 158

SPECT (single photon emission computed tomography), 106, 110–11, 254
sphygmomanometer, 122, 254
sports. *See* exercise; young athletes; *specific sports*
sports drinks, 41
sports podiatrists, 47
spouses/partners
  death of, 70
  supportiveness of, 73, 74
squash, 43
SSRIs. *See* selective serotonin reuptake
  inhibitors
stair stepping, 47
starches, 62, 63
starvation, 177, 178
statins, 7, 135, 152, 231, 254
stem cell therapy, 228, 232–36, 254
stenosis, 254
  tricuspid, 255
  valvular, 147, 150, 200
stent-grafts, 223
stents, 221–22
  air travel and, 207
  angioplasty and placement of, 34,
    112–13, 132–33
  coronary artery disease and, 131–33,
    134
  definition of, 254
  drug-eluting, 173, 221, 222, 250
  high blood pressure and, 127
  women and, 173
step aerobics, 43, 47
stethoscopes, 101, 122, 138, 151
stomach bands/stomach stapling. *See*
  bariatric surgery
strength training, 36, 40, 45
stress
  anger and, 70
  definition of, 69–70
  diet/exercise regimen success and
    reduction of, 32, 51, 73
  family dynamics and, 72–73
  heart attack and, 11, 70

heart failure and, 141
  as heart risk factor, 5, 11–12, 70
  high blood pressure and, 11, 123
  hormones and, 11, 70, 78, 127
  indicators of, 71–72
  management of, 3, 73–76
  shortness of breath and, 17
  smoking and, 10
  women and, 172
stress inoculation therapy. *See* anger
  management training
stress tests. *See* exercise stress tests;
  nuclear stress tests
stretching, 36, 40, 44, 48
stroke
  African Americans and, 187
  baby aspirin prevention of, 173, 174
  cholesterol levels and, 6
  depression and, 78
  embolic, 145
  high blood pressure and, 122
  high-CRP level and, 14
  Native Americans and, 190
  patent foramen ovale and, 223
  risk factors for, 3–8, 10, 14
  smoking and, 10, 82
  women and, 4, 170, 171
stroke volume, exercise and, 32
subvalvular pulmonic stenosis, 254
subvalvular stenosis, 200
subvalvular/supravalvular aortic stenosis, 254
sudden cardiac death
  high CRP level and, 14
  men and, 4
  phobic disorders and, 80, 81
  sleep apnea and, 15
  smoking and, 10
  women and, 80, 195
  young athletes and, 192, 193–95,
    197, 224
  See also cardiac arrest
sugar, 61, 62
sunflower oil, 61

support socks/stockings, 38, 208, 209
supravalvular stenosis, 200
supraventricular arrhythmias, 203, 207, 225
supraventricular tachycardia, 254
surgery, 95, 127
    bariatric, 58–59
    bypass. *See* coronary bypass surgery
    congenital heart disease and, 202, 203
    coronary artery disease and, 131–34, 218
    elderly patients and, 180, 183–84
    heart failure and, 140–41
    heart-valve disorders and, 152–53, 220, 224
    open-heart, 133, 218, 220
    preventive antibiotic therapy and, 152
    recent advances in, 218–21
    robotic, 220
surgical tubing, resistance training and, 36, 47
surgical ventricular restoration, 218–19, 254
swelling (edema), 19, 101, 250
swimming, 12, 35, 40, 43, 47
syncope. *See* fainting
systolic blood pressure, 3, 122, 181
    definition of, 254

tachyarrhythmias, 143, 225, 226
tachycardia, 255
    ventricular, 225, 226
tadalafil, 163
tai chi, 12, 74
"talking pace," 44
tar, 86
tea, 56
    green, 158
    herbal, 162
TEE (transesophageal echocardiography), 111–12
tennis, 38, 43
tetralogy of Fallot, 255
Therabands, 36, 47

therapeutic massage, 158
throat cancer, 87
thrombus, 255
tilt-table testing, 114–15
timolol, 145
tinctures, 162
tobacco. *See* smoking
tonsils, removal of, 15
tooth loss, 87
topical herbal preparations, 162–63
track and field, 38
trainers, 47
tranquilizers, 211
transcendental meditation, 74
transdermal, 255
transesophageal echocardiography, 111–12
transfatty acids, 6, 56
transmyocardial laser revascularization, 220–21, 255
transplants, heart, 140–41, 183–84, 219
transposition of the great arteries, 255
transtelephonic ECGs, 143
travelers, 168, 206–12
    air travel concerns of, 206–9
    drugs and medical records for, 209–10
    exercise and, 36, 41, 47, 210–12
    local doctor recommendations for, 22, 210
treatment plan. *See* individualized treatment program
treatments, 95–96, 120–53
    alternative and complementary therapies, 154–64
    biologically based therapies, 228–38
    clinical trials, 230, 234, 239–43
    device and procedure advances, 215–27
    minority population considerations, 190–91
    women and differences in, 173–74
    young athletes and, 197
    See also specific diseases and conditions

tricuspid atresia, 255
tricuspid regurgitation, 149, 255
tricuspid stenosis, 255
tricuspid valve, 147, 152
triglycerides
    cardiovascular risk and, 7, 8, 135
    definition of, 255
    exercise reduction of, 31
    metabolic syndrome and, 8
    testing for, 101
tropical oils, 6, 56, 61
truncus arteriosus, 255
tumors, 127, 129
type I diabetes, 8
type II diabetes, 8, 9, 31

ultrasound, 127
    cardiac. See resting echocardiography
    Doppler, 108, 119
    intravascular, 113
    vascular, 118
urine tests, 101–3

VADs (ventricular assist devices), 140,
    219–20
vagus nerve, 18
Valium, 87
valve. See aortic valve; heart-valve
    disease; mitral valve; pulmonary valve
valve replacement surgery, 140, 153, 224
valvular dilation, 200
valvular insufficiency, 150
valvular stenosis, 147, 150, 200
varenafil, 163
variables, definition of, 255
varicose veins, 19, 38, 208
vascular endothelial growth factor, 230,
    231, 255
vascular ultrasound, 118
vasculogenesis, 229, 231
vasoconstriction, 255
vasodilators
    definition/function of, 127, 255
    for heart failure, 190

for heart-valve disease, 151–52
for high blood pressure, 139
vectors, 237–38
vegetables, 61, 63, 68
vegetarian diets, 61, 65
VEGF (vascular endothelial growth
    factor), 220, 231, 255
veins, 121
    varicose, 19, 38, 208
venous thrombosis, 255
ventricles, 142, 147, 181
    definition/function of, 255
    double outlet, 250
    surgical restoration of, 140
ventricular arrhythmias, 203, 207
ventricular assist device (VAD), 140,
    219–20, 255
ventricular fibrillation, 145, 193, 255
ventricular remodeling, 233
ventricular septal defect, 200, 255
ventricular tachycardia, 225, 226
verapamil, 145
very-low fat diet, 64
Viagra, 163
viral infection, 13, 136, 194
vision loss, 122
vitamin A, 158
vitamin D, 158
vitamin E, 155
vitamins, 14, 156
    high-dose, 155, 158
Voight, Deborah, 58
vomiting, during exercise, 46

walking, 32, 35, 36, 40, 41, 43, 47
    shoes for, 37–38
warfarin, 145
warm-ups, exercise, 4, 40
warning signs and symptoms, 2, 15–20
    during exercise, 34, 46, 47
    women and, 4, 169, 173
water aerobics, 29, 35
water consumption
    during air travel, 208, 209

diet and, 56
exercise and, 40–41
water pills. *See* diuretics
weather, as exercise consideration, 47
"weekend warriors," 39
weight-bearing exercise, 32
weight-lifting, 43, 197
weight loss and control, 53–65
   comparison of popular diets for, 64
   diet control tips for, 55–57
   differing approaches to, 59–65
   drugs and supplements for, 58
   exercise and, 45, 60
   Food Guide Pyramid and, 55, 63, 65
   heart failure and, 141
   high blood pressure and, 50, 123
   surgical treatments for, 58–59
   See also obesity; overweight
weight training, 45, 48, 49, 182
Weight Watchers, 60, 61, 64
Weil, Andrew, 154
Wellbutrin, 87
white-coat hypertension, 99
whole grains, 61, 68
Wilderness Medical Society, 212
wine, benefits of, 65–66, 158
withdrawal, nicotine, 86, 87, 90
women
   anxiety disorders and, 80–81
   body fat distribution in, 10, 171
   breast cancer worries of, 4–5, 169
   chest-pain sensation in, 4
   cholesterol and, 171
   coronary artery disease and, 4, 172
   depression and, 77, 172
   diabetes and, 170, 171
   diagnostic tests/procedures and, 107, 110, 172
   eating disorders and, 167, 177–78
   exercise and, 49, 170
   fertility problems and, 83, 178
   heart attack and, 4–5, 80, 170, 171, 173, 175

   heart disease and, 4–5, 19–20, 77, 167, 169–78
   heart failure and, 181
   heart risk factors for, 4–5, 7–8, 169, 170
   high blood pressure and, 7–8, 170, 171, 174–75
   hormone replacement therapy and, 4, 170–71, 208
   low-dose aspirin regimen and, 173–74
   menopause and, 4, 10, 83, 171
   menstrual cycle and, 172
   menstrual problems and, 178
   obesity and, 170, 188
   oral contraceptives and, 170
   pregnancy and. *See* pregnancy
   psychological and social issues and, 171–72
   smoking and, 11, 83, 170
   stress and, 172
   stroke and, 4, 170, 171
   sudden cardiac death and, 80, 195
   treatment differences for, 173–74
   warning signs/symptoms for, 4, 169, 173
   weight training and, 45, 49
Women's Health Initiative Study, 4, 171
World Health Organization, 179
wrinkles, smoking and, 83

yoga, 74, 154, 158
yohimbe/yohimbine, 157, 163
young athletes, 167, 192–98
   "athlete's heart" and, 197
   cardiac death causes for, 193–95, 224
   individual variables for, 197
   recommendations concerning, 196
   screening of, 195–96
yo-yo dieting, 57, 68
Yusuf, Salim, 11

Zoloft, 87
Zone diet, 64
Zyban, 87